To Kelli, Sam, and Adam

AND

*To **All** the children I have taught and learned from*

ACKNOWLEDGEMENTS

The following people were instrumental in the development and publication of this book:

The professionals who reviewed and provided vital feedback on the initial manuscript: David Allaway, Valerie Banks, Susan Dukehart, Donna Gibson, M.S.,R.D., Carolyn Johnson, Sheila Lederer, Terri Lloyd-Jones, M.S., R.D., and Gordon McDonald, CWC.

The children who tested (and tasted!) many of the edible art activities: Kate Boudreau, James Case, Marit Case, Kelli Evers, Jacob Fitzgerald, Mackenzie Miller, and Robert Stewart.

Students of Portland Public Schools who wrote funny, endearing, and often revealing thank-you letters over the years, some of which are excerpted in the quotes that begin each chapter.

My editor, Cheri Swoboda, CFCS, for her valuable suggestions and much-needed reassurance.

Carol Buckle, graphic designer and friend who, in addition to her marvelous design, cover art, and illustrations, managed to keep me in good humor.

The Tigard Public Library staff, for their tireless assistance in helping me locate books, reference materials, and resources.

Brenda Ponichtera, R.D., author/publisher of the best selling *Quick & Healthy* cookbooks, who provided invaluable advice, encouragement, and mentoring.

And finally, to my husband Scott, and children Kelli, Sam, and Adam, for their love and understanding, and to my parents, Gus and Shirley Liakos, for their enduring encouragement and support.

What Reviewers and Readers Are Saying About...

HOW TO TEACH NUTRITION TO KIDS

"...an excellent resource for those in the position of teaching nutrition to children..."
– *Journal of the American Dietetic Association*

"...essential reading for parents, teachers, school nutritionists, and anyone who influences the nutritional values of today's youth."
– *School Food Service RESEARCH REVIEW*

"...one of the most creative books you'll find on nutrition or on activities in any of the discipline areas. *Outstanding*."
– *Teaching K-8, The Professional Ideabook for Teachers*

"...innovative, imaginative, practical, and effective!"
– *The Midwest Book Review*

"Parents, as well as teachers, will find a lot of fun, hands-on activities in this book."
– *The Oregonian*

"Evers' philosophy is to keep nutrition education child-centered. In her book, she offers dozens of activities for both teachers and parents to empower kids to make good choices."
– *The Chicago Tribune*

"Evers writes well, employing a brisk style that makes everything clear without being simplistic.... This book holds out the opportunity for parents and schools to cooperate in helping children develop healthy eating and exercise habits."
– *The Statesman Journal (Salem, OR)*

"A must-have book for teachers!"
– *Teachers' Edition Online*

"...delightful and so helpful, just filled with great, usable ideas... a great contribution to those of us that teach."
– *Iowa youth nutrition leader*

"...your writing is wonderful; and I've certainly promoted your book to health educators in our state..."
– *Missouri dietitian*

"...189 pages of fun and exciting nutrition education activities and strategies.... The lessons are child-based, so kids are engaged and learning actively."
– *Food-Net Newsletter*

"I would like to compliment you on your book. I've been recommending it to everyone!"
– *State Nutrition Education & Training (NET) Coordinator*

24 Carrot Press
P.O. Box 23546
Tigard, OR 97281-3546
503-524-9318

Cover, Design, & Illustration: Carol Buckle Design+Illustration
Typesetting: William H. Brunson, Typography Services
Editing: Cheri Swoboda, CFCS

Printed in the United States of America
First Printing – August 1995   Third Printing – October 1997
Second Printing – April 1996

Library of Congress Catalog Card Number 95-90600

Publisher's Cataloging in Publication

Evers, Connie Liakos
    How to teach nutrition to kids : an integrated, creative approach to nutrition education for children ages 6-10.
        p. cm.
    Includes bibliographical references and index.
    Preassigned LCCN: 95-90600.
    ISBN 0-9647970-3-8

    1. Nutrition—Study and teaching.   2. Children—Nutrition.   I. Title

TX364.E84 1995   613.2'083
                                                             QBI95-20419

TABLE OF CONTENTS

INTRODUCTION

Food is an integral part of life. From our first suckling of the breast until our very last meal, food never lingers far from our minds or activities. Food brings people together—for daily meals, wedding feasts, backyard cook-outs, sporting events, and just about every social occasion imaginable.

In other words, food goes way beyond nutrition. Nutrition pertains to the myriad of chemical reactions that occur inside the body. From the combustion of carbohydrate for energy to the healing of a paper cut to the building of bone in a growing child, nutrition in action is something we don't have to consciously think about.

But to supply the best raw materials for the elegant workings of our body, we must give food some thought. Eating habits and food memories are imprinted early on and difficult to change later, a fact many adults learn all too well when they attempt to alter life-long eating behaviors.

The purpose of this book is to give educators, nutrition professionals, parents, and other caregivers the tools they need to teach 6-10 year-old children about nutrition in a meaningful and integrated way. Ideas are drawn from my experience as a nutrition educator in a large urban school district and my job as a parent feeding three children. Along the way, I have learned a great deal about how to succeed in teaching nutrition to kids. I have also had a lot of fun doing it! I hope you share my enthusiasm and allow your own creativity to expand and build on the many ideas presented here.

HOW TO USE THIS BOOK

A cooperative approach among caregivers is necessary if children are to both learn and practice good eating habits. Described below are suggestions on how those who care for and teach children can best incorporate ideas and activities from this book.

Educators

The chapters in this book bare little resemblance to a standard nutrition book. Take a look at the Table of Contents. Instead of chapters like "Vegetables," "Vitamins," or "Food Labels," you will see "Language Arts," "Math," and "Social Studies," the subjects teachers spend time on every day of the school year! Many of the lesson ideas are designed with time in mind—easy to implement with little preparation. Others can be modified for simplicity or expanded into a comprehensive unit. (The gardening ideas in Chapter 7 could easily comprise a year-long theme!).

Throughout this book, you can readily identify how nutrition lesson ideas crossover into other disciplines. The following picture symbols identify related subject areas:

 Language Arts   Math   Science   Social Studies

 Performing Arts   Art   Physical Education   Cafeteria

Activities that require materials and supplies beyond what is commonly found in most classrooms are highlighted with **"You Will Need"** boxes. Activities and books are categorized according to level (primary, intermediate, or either) in the index listing for each subject area.

Chapter 4, "Teaching The Basics: The Food Guide Pyramid," provides guidance on how to design your introductory nutrition unit, ideally taught early in the school year. Once students have a grasp of these basic concepts, you can expand and reinforce nutrition by integrating it into your curriculum—all year long! As you plan your units of instruction and learning centers, keep this book handy. Refer to each subject area chapter as you plan lessons.

Many of the nutrition ideas may be the hook to get kids motivated in other subjects, too. Writing a letter to "Baby Bear," graphing food intake, or analyzing the school lunch menu can make writing, math, and critical thinking more exciting and relevant.

Before you plan lessons involving food preparation, please review Appendix A, "Guidelines For Safe Classroom Cooking."

Finally, take a look around your classroom. Are food and nutrition teaching materials up-to-date? If you have a kitchen, grocery store or restaurant as part of your dramatic play area, do the play foods include healthful choices? (An inexpensive way to update this area is to use real food packages, stuffed with pillow foam, if needed.) Do you still have posters of the old "four food groups?" (Or the really old four food groups, the one with butter in the dairy group?)

Resources for low-cost materials that will brighten your classroom and reinforce nutrition concepts are listed in Appendix B.

Food/Nutrition Professionals

Just as nutrition is integrated into all subject areas, this book also gives guidance for integrating nutrition education into the school meal program. After all, the school cafeteria is the ultimate laboratory, giving students the chance to practice nutrition concepts each day!

In nearly every chapter, students are encouraged to become involved with the school nutrition program. Examples include touring the school kitchen, writing letters to the school nutrition director, analyzing the school breakfast and lunch menus, and performing lunchtime nutrition skits.

Whenever possible, make yourself available to the teachers and students in your school. Volunteer to be a guest speaker on nutrition. Your presentation can be as simple as reading a storybook with a good-food message or as complicated as setting up a classroom sandwich bar to illustrate a meal that exemplifies the *Food Guide Pyramid*. This book provides hundreds of ideas on classroom nutrition lessons.

Another powerful way to reinforce nutrition concepts is to run promotions in the cafeteria. Menu or recipe contests, food-of-the-week displays, nutrition bingo with small incentives, student poster art, and point-of-choice nutrition information encourage students to make healthful food choices. Chapter 12 provides guidance on how to turn the cafeteria into a center for nutrition education.

Parents

You are the ultimate gatekeeper of nutrition. What you buy, how you cook, the foods that you eat or refuse—all send strong messages about food to your child. The best way to educate your child about nutrition and health is to model good eating behavior.

Beyond your role as food provider and living example, there are many other ways to teach your child about food and nutrition. A number of ideas in this book can easily be adapted for learning situations in the home. Tending a small garden plot, reading and discussing books with nutrition messages, or using the grocery store as a learning center are just a few examples.

Involve your child in the kitchen. It's true that cooking with your child may add to the time, mess, and confusion initially. But eventually, you will appreciate both the extra set of hands and your child's growing self-sufficiency.

Many of the food activities, especially the edible art creations in Chapter 10, work well in group settings such as birthday parties, scout meetings, or large family gatherings.

This book can also serve as a stepping stone for initiating a nutrition education program in your local elementary school. Activities and ideas can be implemented by parent volunteers in the classroom or at school wellness, health, multicultural, or science fairs. Information presented here also provides valuable guidance for setting school nutrition policy.

CHAPTER 1

MAKING THE CASE FOR NUTRITION EDUCATION

"I want to learn all about nutrition. Because my Grandpa had a heart attack and had to have heart bypass surgery. When we got to see him he had lots of tubes in him. So I hope I stay healthy."–Erin

A Great Need

The message of good nutrition is not reaching the youngest and most vulnerable members of our society, at least not in a meaningful way. Current findings shed a dim light on the state of children's eating and exercise habits.

KIDS AT RISK An estimated 40 percent of school-aged children already possess at least one risk factor for heart disease, including obesity, high blood pressure, or high blood cholesterol. Children as young as five who are overweight and inactive tend to have higher blood pressure than their more active peers. Fatty streaks, the first stage of buildup in the arteries that eventually leads to blockage and heart attacks, are often well-established by the end of the teen-age years.

INACTIVITY Even while studies point to a decline in calorie and fat intake in the past decade, today's children are fatter than ever. Obesity now affects 27% of children and 21% of the teens in this country, an increase of 54% and 39%, respectively, since the 1970's. It is estimated that about half of overfat school-agers will remain obese into adulthood.

A big contributor to this trend is our entrance into the "video age," with kids spending large chunks of passive time in front of the television, video games, and computers. Studies have documented a clear connection between the time spent watching TV and the levels of both body fat and blood cholesterol in kids.

Besides increasing the temptation to snack on advertised foods, television has replaced active play for many kids. In a recent survey, 22 percent of children ages six to nine said they seldom play outside, even when the weather is nice. In contrast, 80 percent reported they watch television after school and on Saturdays.

POOR FOOD CHOICES With a food supply as plentiful and varied as we have in the U.S., it is shocking to note the dismal state of children's (and adult's!) food choices. According to government statistics, a mere 9% of 6-11 year-old children eat the recommended five servings of fruits and vegetables each day. (Only 25% of adults get their "five-a-day.")

A recent survey of New York second and fifth graders found that on a typical day, 15% of the children ate *no* vegetables and 20% ate *no* fruit. Sixteen percent of the fifth graders skipped breakfast. The children's favorite snack foods were cookies, ice cream, soft drinks, chips, and candy.

Only one in three third through twelfth graders report eating the right kinds of food very often, according to the Kellogg Children's Nutrition Survey, which polled more than 5000 children nationwide. Pop, cupcakes, cookies, and candy edged out fruit and vegetable consumption while beef, pork, hot dogs, and hamburgers were eaten more often than lower fat turkey, chicken, or fish.

Few youngsters take in enough calcium to maximize their lifetime bone development. At a time when they need calcium the most, kids are choosing soft drinks over dairy products and potato chips over broccoli. While recent government recommendations advise a calcium intake of 800-1200 milligrams for children ages 6-10, nutrition surveys show a decline in calcium intake for this age group, with fewer than half consuming 800 milligrams each day.

HUNGRY CHILDREN Poverty impacts the diets of a startling number of children in America. According to data from the Food Research and Action Center, there are 5½ million children in this country who do not get enough to eat. Another 6 million are at risk for hunger due to poverty.

Hungry children often fail to achieve their full academic potential. Children with inadequate diets are sick more, less active, less able to think and concentrate, and more irritable and anxious. Kids with iron deficiency anemia score lower on IQ tests (especially in vocabulary), and suffer from perceptual difficulties and low achievement.

One partial solution to this problem is better promotion of the school breakfast and lunch programs. Children who eat school meals, regardless of income level, have higher intakes of key nutrients and perform better in school.

Opportunity For Change

The news about children's nutrition is not all bad. On the upside, a tremendous amount of interest, effort and opportunity currently surrounds this problem.

CONCERNED PARENTS In spite of time demands and financial pressures, parents are increasingly concerned about their children's health and fitness. When The Post Center for Nutrition and Health surveyed consumers in order to identify the top 100 questions Americans most want answered about nutrition as it relates to their health, the number one question was *"What foods are best for children to eat?"* Seventh on the list was *"How does a lot of sugar affect children?"* while the question *"How do you get children to eat properly?"* was rated eighth.

Parents still have considerable influence over the eating patterns of their children. Studies point to a strong association between parents who model good nutrition and improved eating habits in their youngsters. School-based nutrition programs that involve parents are more effective at changing children's eating behaviors than those that focus solely on the student.

KIDS IN THE KITCHEN As children become more self-reliant at an earlier age, a "teachable moment" exists for strengthening food-related life skills. Children are increasingly the caretakers of their own nutrition. A 1991 Gallup survey found that 87 percent of the fourth through eighth graders sampled said that they cook or make some of their own meals. Eighty-three percent said they sometimes prepare their own snacks and eight out of ten sometimes cook or make their own breakfast. Surprisingly, more than half of the kids surveyed actually buy the food for their own meals or snacks.

Children who don't know how to cook often rely on packaged foods of questionable nutritional quality. For this growing number of young consumers, nutrition education can really work when concepts are practical and applied, emphasizing skills like shopping, label reading, and cooking. Kids who are on their own for meals can immediately translate their nutrition knowledge into healthy eating behavior.

SCHOOL MEAL REFORM Schools participating in the United States Department of Agriculture (USDA) child nutrition program will see sweeping program reforms in the next few years. Students will see more healthful fare on their breakfast and lunch trays as schools fully implement the *Dietary Guidelines for Americans* set forth by USDA (See Chapter 12). With the implementation of the new regulations, school nutrition providers will increasingly play a role in the nutrition education of students.

CHANGES IN EDUCATION One goal of *Healthy People 2000*, the set of federal objectives for health promotion released in 1990, is to "increase to at least 75 percent the proportion of the Nation's schools that provide nutrition education from preschool through 12th grade, preferably as part of quality school health education."

At present, fewer than one-fourth of states require nutrition education in school while few colleges and universities include nutrition coursework as part of the core curriculum for elementary teachers.

But with the realization that well-nourished students learn better, elementary teachers are becoming more inclined to move beyond the basic food groups and teach nutrition in a comprehensive, behavior-oriented manner. As integrated education takes hold, teachers will increasingly seek ways to infuse nutrition across the curriculum.

A Call To Action

Clearly, the efforts of many are needed to reverse the trends set forth in this chapter. The messages children receive about nutrition should be clear, consistent, and constant. Only then will they begin to internalize the information and make changes in their eating and activity. This formidable task of presenting these messages is shared by all who influence kids' food choices: parents, extended family, educators, food/nutrition professionals, health care providers, researchers, the food industry, the media, and politicians.

Most importantly, the food available to children must match the message they are hearing. Whether at school, home, the ballpark, or a restaurant, healthful choices that appeal to kids are essential. Kids don't get proficient at playing the piano, solving math problems, or scoring soccer goals without a lot of practice—the same is true of good nutrition habits!

CHAPTER 2

THE MESSAGE OF HEALTHY EATING

"I enjoyed you coming in and telling us about how we should eat better food. And that healthy food can taste good too. I'm fat, so I should take your advice."–Ten

Finding a Balance

MEDIA MESSAGES Presenting a balanced picture of nutrition is no easy task in today's society. The media scares us daily, reporting the latest nutrition study as fact, leaving us dazed as we contemplate whether our favorite foods have been praised or denounced this week. We quickly lose sight that food really is enjoyable and necessary and sustains our life!

Likewise, children are sent a mind-boggling set of mixed messages from television and print media. On one hand, they see mostly "beautiful" people—at least by Hollywood or Madison Avenue's standard—who are thin, rich, popular, and fun-loving. On the other hand, they are barraged with advertisements for junk food. When they do see the beautiful people eating, it is usually for ads that peddle pop, chips, candy, or ice cream!

Long before they can read or write, children are influenced by advertising messages. In addition to the 30,000 TV ads each year aimed at kids, companies also reach children through in-school promotions, Kids' Clubs, cross-selling and other promotions, according to a report published by Consumer Union.

Licensing Barbie to sell breakfast cereal, watching popular stars drink Pepsi and Coke, offering a Kids' Club at Burger King, and featuring Domino's pizza in Teenage Mutant Ninja Turtles movies are examples of food promotions that make a big impression on children.

When the Center for Science in the Public Interest studied Saturday morning programming on ABC, NBC, CBS, the Fox network, and Nickelodeon cable channel, they found that 222 of the 340 ads in a given morning were for foods. A measly eight of the batch were for "reasonably nutritious" products such as low-sugar breakfast cereals, frozen entrees and milk, while the rest centered on foods with a low nutrient profile.

Adding to the confusion, many ads directed at kids are deceptive in their nature. For instance, breakfast cereals with "fruit" or "fruity" in their name are depicted in ads that include colorful images of real fruit. In reality, many of the products contain no fruit or juice, relying on artificial flavors and colors for their "fruitiness."

Unfortunately, it appears that kids are taking these pitches to heart. With over $1 billion dollars a week in buying power (including the purchases they influence as well as ones they make themselves), the top food purchases of children include candy and gum, soft drinks, snacks and fast food.

ALTERED BODY IMAGE Not only is our society getting fatter, we also feel more guilty about it, a feeling children are acquiring at an alarmingly young age. Over 60 percent of fourth grade girls in an Iowa study reported a desire to be thinner. By age 18, nine out of ten teen-age girls in a California survey were dieting to lose weight.

This perception of fatness is common even among girls with little body fat. In one study, 58% of girls ages 9 to 18 thought of themselves as fat, whereas only 15% were overfat based on height and weight measures. Fear of fatness, restrained eating, and binge eating were found to be common among girls by age 10.

Boys may also have a disturbed body image, but their orientation is toward a bigger and more muscular physique.

Parents have a powerful influence on their children's self-esteem and body image. In one study, measured self-esteem scores of kids ages 9-11 were lowered when they thought their parents were dissatisfied with their bodies. In boys, a lowered self-esteem was linked with both thinness and being perceived as too thin by parents. Not surprisingly, lowered self esteem in girls had more to do with parental attitudes toward fatness.

Adding to the image problem is a small but worrisome group of overzealous parents. Determined that their child will not be fat or eat fat, they restrict food intake starting at a very young age. Kids who comply with their parents wishes often end up underweight and at risk for delayed growth. Those who rebel may end up overweight because they have a tendency to overeat whenever they get the chance.

There is a wide variation in growth patterns and rates among kids. Children of the same age can vary as much as 40 pounds and 10 inches and still be considered "normal" by growth standards. Unfortunately, kids don't see a wide variety of shapes and sizes depicted in magazines or television. Even their school textbooks carry a "size-bias." An analysis of third-grade texts since the beginning of the century found that illustrations of girls became increasingly thinner through the years while no change was noted for pictures of boys.

Creating Positive Attitudes

Reversing the trend of feeling guilty about food and weight, resulting in indulgence, more weight, and more guilt, can only be arrested through education and self awareness.

If we are to instill healthy attitudes about food and body image in our children, we must start early, presenting a unified message about food as friend and bodies as something to be proud and happy about.

Now the hard part—we, as adult role models, must reach some degree of satisfaction with ourselves! Women, in particular, spend enormous time and energy pursuing that elusive ideal of a "perfect" body. In our constant obsession to diet, exercise, and sometimes—engage in dubious weight loss practices—we often forget that our basic body shape was predetermined at birth!

It's no wonder we're confused. In our lifetime alone, we have seen the "ideal" female body form go from the voluptuous Marilyn Monroe to rail-thin Twiggy.

While the 90's have seen more emphasis on muscular models, we have also seen a return of emaciation as beauty, known in the popular press as the "waif-look."

WHAT WE CAN DO Despite the influence of popular culture, there are steps we can take to instill healthy attitudes in our children:

• Affirm children. When they complain about being too fat, skinny, short, tall, or slow, emphasize the goodness about them. Assure them that people—that means kids, too—come in all different colors, shapes, and sizes. There is no one "best" way to look.

A helpful resource on this subject is the book *Am I Fat? Helping Young Children Accept Differences in Body Size*, by Joanne Ikeda and Priscilla Naworski (See Appendix B).

• Children who you suspect are overfat should be referred to a qualified health care provider for evaluation and treatment. Often, counseling of an obese child requires cooperation and participation by the entire family and school community.

• Emphasize the enjoyable aspects of food. Avoid labeling food as either medicine or poison. With older children especially, telling them "it's good for you" may be the kiss of death for a particular food. Likewise, kids are not immediately concerned that a food they like may clog their arteries or decay their teeth. Scare tactics rarely work.

• Children should have a choice over their eating and control over their bodies. Given a selection of healthful foods, kids have an amazing ability to regulate their diet. In spite of good intentions, adults often throw children's eating habits out of whack when they attempt to regulate food intake.

Taken to extreme, an over-controlling parent places a child at risk for developing eating disorders such as obesity, bulimia, and anorexia nervosa.

A must-read on this subject is Ellyn Satter's *How to Get Your Kid to Eat ... But Not Too Much* (See Appendix B).

• Encourage children to move, play, and exercise, both at home and at school. Besides physical education and recess time, kids (and teachers!) can benefit from discovery classroom walks (see Chapter 11).

At home, kids will gravitate toward more activity if they are regularly "unplugged" from television and video games. Parents also reap benefits from family walks, bike rides, and other shared activities.

• Make family meals a priority. Breaking bread together promotes good nutrition habits. School-aged children who eat alone in front of the television tend to overeat, while younger children tend to eat fewer nutritious foods when isolated at meals.

Mealtime means more than refueling kids with nutrients—they also get a hefty dose of emotional, intellectual, and spiritual nourishment. As families pass the peas and pour the milk, they also convey values and establish traditions.

Pay attention to the school mealtime atmosphere, too. Bright cafeterias, short lines, and adequate time for children to eat should be goals of every school. Kids should be allowed to relax and socialize—those skills contribute to learning, too! Schools with limited facilities may want to explore "family-style" eating in the classroom.

What Kids Need to Know

Clearly, children are in desperate need of a balanced, sensible message about eating and nutrition. One goal of nutrition education is to enlighten and empower kids so that they will grow to be adults who make informed food choices, avoiding the lure of the latest "food fright."

What then, should we be teaching kids? The following points outline the basic goals of nutrition education for kids. Chapters 4-12 provide specific, hands-on activities for reaching these goals.

• Emphasize food as it relates to life today. You will lose kids' attention faster than they can say "osteoporosis" if too much emphasis is placed on how proper nutrition prevents disease. If you succeed in reaching them with the good nutrition message today, their tomorrows will likely be healthier too.

Remind children that healthful food promotes achievement. In school or on the playing field, kids who eat well perform better and achieve higher levels of mastery. A nutritious diet fuels the body for learning, growth, sports, and play.

Well-nourished kids look better, too! Children who eat a balanced diet have bright, sparkly eyes, healthy skin, hair, and teeth, and bodies that look and feel great.

• The message of good nutrition is summed up in the first six *Dietary Guidelines for Americans*. Adults and kids over the age of two are advised to eat from a wide selection of foods, emphasize grains, fruits and vegetables, moderate the amount of fat, sugar, and sodium they eat, and keep their weight in check. Simple advice that's often hard to put into practice!

Dietary Guidelines for Americans

U.S. Department of Agriculture/ U.S. Department of Health & Human Services, fourth edition, 1995.

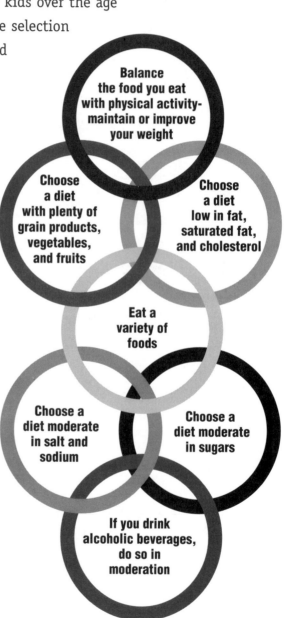

Balance the food you eat with physical activity- maintain or improve your weight

Choose a diet with plenty of grain products, vegetables, and fruits

Choose a diet low in fat, saturated fat, and cholesterol

Eat a variety of foods

Choose a diet moderate in salt and sodium

Choose a diet moderate in sugars

If you drink alcoholic beverages, do so in moderation

Two important practical tools for meeting these guidelines are the *Food Guide Pyramid* and the *Nutrition Facts* food label. A "picture" of what a healthful diet looks like, the pyramid is especially useful as a teaching aid for children. The revised food label is a simplified, yet effective, device for analyzing foods and comparing their nutrient content. Ideas for developing a nutrition unit around the *Food Guide Pyramid* and nutrition labels are included, respectively, in chapters four and six.

• Teach children to refuel their bodies! Because of their smaller stomach capacity and tremendous energy needs, kids require frequent meals and snacks. Behavior problems at times are merely the result of an empty stomach.

Somehow, "snacking" has taken on a negative connotation in our society, perhaps because it is often linked with junk food. Done right, snacks can and do make a big contribution to daily nutrition. Healthful snacks should mirror meals—emphasizing healthful foods, but in smaller quantities.

Breakfast is the meal most directly connected to school achievement. Kids who skip breakfast have shorter attention spans, do poorly in tasks requiring concentration, and even score lower on standard achievement tests.

When researchers compared the diets of children who regularly eat breakfast with those who don't, they found that the breakfast skippers never fully compensate for the missed meal throughout the day. Children who ate a morning meal took in far more nutrients over the course of the day than those who missed breakfast.

• Young bodies need to move! Nutrition studies show that the increasing problem of childhood obesity stems more from inactivity than overeating. An intricate balance exists between food and physical activity. A nutrition unit will be decidedly lacking if it fails to present the exercise part of the equation. Kids enjoy learning about nutrition when it is presented from a fitness perspective. That's why Chapter 11 is devoted to nutrition as part of the physical education curriculum. Physical fitness should also be part of the daily classroom routine, especially in schools that limit PE to once or twice weekly.

• If children are to resist the allure of the media, advertisements, and other societal influences, they must learn to identify the intent of the messages. Even very young children can grasp the basic purpose of advertising (to sell us stuff!). Older children will enjoy homework they really can do in front of the T.V., i.e. analyze and critique food ads!

Role playing is a very effective way to teach children the messages of the media and encourage the development of critical thinking and decision-making skills. Chapter nine outlines several strategies for helping children to analyze and re-create the food messages they hear each day from TV, radio, magazines, and peers.

CHAPTER 3

THE F.I.B. APPROACH TO NUTRITION EDUCATION

"I had a lot of fun with you. The bread was delicious. I am going to be a bread maker when I grow-up. And I am going to make whole wheat bread—a lot of whole wheat bread."–Angela

Fun, Integrated, and Behavioral

There was little in my training to become a registered dietitian that prepared me to teach nutrition to kids. Those early college years were spent learning the scientific basis of nutrition and key principles of food management. Not that the zinc requirement of rodents or hospital trayline efficiency weren't important issues, it's just that I failed to grasp the practical issues at the heart of feeding kids.

Things like what to do when kids decorated the wall with their spaghetti or called coconuts "dog poop balls" or stuffed peas up their nose.

Or, how to avoid boring kids to sleep with talk of food groups!

As the years progressed, I gained insight from those around me—kids, teachers, parents, and foodservice providers. I came to realize that key elements were often missing from efforts at nutrition education.

Boiled down to three words, the ingredients I discovered necessary for effective nutrition education with children are **Fun**, **Integrated**, and **Behavioral**. Hence the acronym F.I.B. (though I certainly don't advocate lying!).

Make It Fun!

Like it or not, kids in the 90's are easily bored. Products of the video age, they are used to information that is fast-paced and exciting. In a word, "fun."

Teachers increasingly need to engage as well as educate students. While this approach can mean more planning, the payoff is a boost in motivation. Children who enjoy themselves through discovery and experimentation are much more apt to listen and retain information.

Educators who create engaging lessons often enjoy their jobs more, too! During my career as a nutrition educator, I have:

• Appeared in classrooms around Halloween as "Nutra the Witch," teaching kids how to make "food group brew", choose healthy snacks, and limit their candy "goblin."

• Acted in noontime nutrition shows for elementary schools with two full-sized dog characters named Sheggy Good-Grub and Sickly Spot. I even led the cafeteria in "The Sheggy Good-Grub Song," in spite of limited vocal skills (once, it was even broadcast on CNN!)

• Used my own baby as a "visual aid." Frustrated with my inability to reach teen moms, I brought my 10 month-old son along to demonstrate techniques for infant feeding. It was fun and also very effective!

• Sang, danced, exercised, cooked, and led puppet shows with elementary school kids more times than I can count!

THINK BIG When planning a nutrition lesson or entire unit, brainstorm creative ways to make the concepts come alive. Say, for example, kids are routinely feeding their oranges to the trash during lunch. Your goal is to encourage kids to eat (or at least try) oranges.

Talking about oranges is boring. Putting up colorful posters of oranges all throughout the school is a little better. Providing cut up oranges for snacks is better still.

But to really make an impact, declare one day "Orange Day." Serve orange juice on the breakfast menu and orange wedges at lunch. Encourage students, staff, and visiting parents to wear orange, call the citrus commission to see if they have teaching materials (and maybe even an orange costume to lend), and set up centers where students can make orange juice, plant the seeds from their oranges, or write a story about oranges. Ask parents to send favorite recipes using oranges or orange juice. Decorate the cafeteria with student-made "Orange you glad you eat oranges?" posters. The ideas are endless ...

Overkill? Perhaps. But this example illustrates how one nutrition concept—oranges are a good food to eat—can be integrated into the entire school environment. Students pick up skills in science (making orange juice and planting seeds), language arts (writing a story), and art (making posters). Staff, parents, and the school cafeteria all become involved, too, making this an *integrated* effort. Which leads us to the next letter of "F.I.B."

Integrate Nutrition Wherever Possible

Success with nutrition education largely depends on how well it is integrated into other subject areas, intertwined with the school cafeteria, and reinforced through food experiences at home.

With barely enough time to teach kids the "basics," teachers struggle to find time to teach nutrition. It's not that they aren't interested, either. In one survey, 90% of elementary teachers felt that nutrition should be taught in school but only half reported having time for nutrition education.

While teachers prefer to integrate nutrition into other subject areas, they don't always have the time or skills to accomplish this goal. In a Wisconsin survey, thirty percent of elementary school teachers integrate nutrition into their curriculum, but a whopping 76% would prefer this approach. While 23% of the teachers in this survey taught nutrition separately, only a mere 4% actually preferred this method.

Not surprisingly, studies show that when nutrition is an integral part of the school day, teachers teach more nutrition over the course of the year than when they present it as a separate unit.

THE CAFETERIA Once thought of as a necessary distraction, the school nutrition program will play an increasing role in the education of students as new federal guidelines are fully implemented. While they serve kids breakfast and lunch, nutrition staff will also be enlisted to serve good-nutrition messages.

As school nutrition directors redesign menus to meet the *Dietary Guidelines for Americans*, implement new menu planning systems, strive for universal meals, and struggle to meet the nutritional needs of chronically ill children, success will depend on the strength of their integration with the classroom and school community.

To be truly effective, the food and messages received in the school cafeteria should complement nutrition instruction by teachers. A solid nutrition education program in the classroom will confuse and dismay students if they are faced with a display of high-fat, low-nutrient fare in the cafeteria. Likewise, making healthful meal changes without teaching students, parents, and school staff the rationale behind the menu switch will likely result in a lot of grumbling and a drop in cafeteria sales.

Chapter 12 is devoted to making the cafeteria a center for nutrition education.

TAKING THE MESSAGE HOME It is essential to link nutrition education to the home environment. Through parent meetings, interaction with parent-teacher groups, newsletters, menus, and information sent home, good nutrition concepts can be reinforced.

Parents have a lot to contribute, too! Joining their child at school meals, setting up health and nutrition "fairs," assisting with classroom nutrition lessons, volunteering in the school kitchen or cafeteria, or selling *nutritious* foods as a fundraiser for education projects are important ways parents can become involved in school nutrition.

Since the bulk of purchasing, food preparation, and eating happens at home, kids may need to serve as nutrition teachers too, encouraging parents to buy and try new foods and experiment with different cooking methods.

Assigning cooking "homework" is one way to get the family (and maybe even the dog) involved!

Emphasize Behavior Change

Nutrition is not just another "subject." Like health or physical education, the goal reaches beyond the acquisition of knowledge. Ultimately, we want to produce changes in the daily eating behavior of children. As the example above illustrates, knowing oranges are nutritious isn't enough—eating more oranges is the bottom-line goal.

Behavior change does not happen quickly, particularly in adults. It is a process—an evolution that requires a cycle of attempts and failures to finally succeed. That is why smokers quit and start many times before finally quitting. Or those seeking a slimmer figure lose, plateau, gain, and lose weight over and over again.

Fortunately, it is easier to produce nutrition and health behavior change in children. Especially before age 12, children are much more likely to take concepts they learn and put them to practice. In a Minnesota study which tracked children from grade six through adolescence, kids who learned to make positive health decisions in regard to smoking, physical activity, and food choices prior to sixth grade ended up with healthier habits as teens.

However, teaching nutrition once a year as a unit, regardless of intensity, will have little impact on long-term behavior change. Those concepts need to be reinforced all year, for many years, to make appreciable changes.

Lessons aimed at behavior change have two things in common: 1) real experience with food and 2) a real-life, reachable goal.

A lesson about grains might include a bread baking (and eating!) activity and end by encouraging students to eat at least six servings each day. Devising a chart to check-off how many grains are eaten would give students a chance to sharpen math skills. Homework could consist of a simple muffin or granola recipe for the students to try with their family. The school cafeteria might highlight the foods made from grain that week, even including a few new ones such as couscous or quinoa. Again, this is an example of an integrated approach to nutrition education aimed at behavior change (A fun one, too!)

Perhaps the best case for promoting good eating behavior is the immediate effects it has on learning and development. A child who is hungry or poorly nourished is not ready to learn. Nutrition education done right is a boost for education in general. Practicing good nutrition habits makes kids better learners of *all* subjects.

CHAPTER 4

TEACHING THE BASICS: THE FOOD GUIDE PYRAMID

"It was fun when you and (chef) Darrell came into our class and showed us the food pyramid and how to make fun snacks."–Lauren

One way to teach children basic nutrition concepts is to build a unit around the *Food Guide Pyramid*. A very visual tool, the pyramid illustrates the proportions of a healthful diet. With its debut in 1992, the pyramid officially took the place of the "basic four food groups."

While the *Dietary Guidelines for Americans* have long urged us to eat more grains, fruits, vegetables, less fat and sugar, and control our weight, they never quite gave us the specifics for accomplishing these noble goals. The *Food Guide Pyramid* puts the dietary guidelines into a graphic form, complete with recommended amounts, that we can use in planning our daily diets.

Food Guide Pyramid
A Guide to Daily Food Choices.

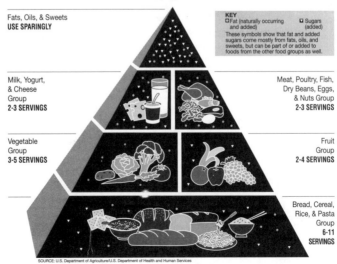

Fats, Oils, & Sweets
USE SPARINGLY

KEY
☐ Fat (naturally occurring and added)   ☐ Sugars (added)
These symbols show that fat and added sugars come mostly from fats, oils, and sweets, but can be part of or added to foods from the other food groups as well.

Milk, Yogurt, & Cheese Group
2-3 SERVINGS

Meat, Poultry, Fish, Dry Beans, Eggs, & Nuts Group
2-3 SERVINGS

Vegetable Group
3-5 SERVINGS

Fruit Group
2-4 SERVINGS

Bread, Cereal, Rice, & Pasta Group
6-11 SERVINGS

SOURCE: U.S. Department of Agriculture/U.S. Department of Health and Human Services

TABLE 4-1

WHAT COUNTS AS ONE SERVING?

Breads, Cereals, Rice and Pasta
1 slice of bread
1/2 cup of cooked rice or pasta
1/2 cup of cooked cereal
1 ounce of ready-to eat cereal

Vegetables
1/2 cup of chopped raw or cooked
   vegetables
1 cup of leafy raw vegetables

Fruits
1 piece of fruit or melon wedge
3/4 cup of juice
1/2 cup of canned fruit
1/4 cup of dried fruit

Milk, Yogurt and Cheese
1 cup of milk or yogurt
1-1/2 to 2 ounces of cheese

Meat, Poultry, Fish, Dry Beans, Eggs and Nuts
2-1/2 to 3 ounces of cooked lean meat,
   poultry or fish
Count 1/2 cup of cooked beans, or 1 egg,
   or 2 tablespoons of peanut butter as 1
   ounce of lean meat (about 1/3 serving)

Fats, Oils and Sweets
LIMIT CALORIES FROM THESE
especially if you need to lose weight

NOTE: The amount you eat may be more than one serving. For example, a dinner portion of spaghetti would count as two or three servings of pasta. Source: USDA/USDHHS

TABLE 4-2

HOW MANY SERVINGS DO YOU NEED EACH DAY?

	Women & some older adults	Children, teen girls active women, most men	Teen boys & active men
Calorie level*	about 1,600	about 2,200	about 2,800
Bread group	6	9	11
Vegetable group	3	4	5
Fruit group	2	3	4
Milk group	**2–3	**2–3	**2–3
Meat group	2, for a total of 5 ounces	2, for a total of 6 ounces	3, for a total of 7 ounces

These are the calorie levels if you choose lowfat, lean foods from the 5 major food groups and use foods from the fats, oils and sweets group sparingly.

**Woman who are pregnant or breastfeeding, teenagers, and young adults to age 24 need 3 servings.* Source: USDA/USDHHS

The Food Guide Pyramid as Teaching Tool

Before you begin your unit, order some of the free and low-cost *Food Guide Pyramid* materials suggested in Appendix B. At the very least, obtain a classroom-sized poster from either the National Livestock & Meat Board or Consumer Information Center.

NOTE: In order to simplify the somewhat cumbersome names given the food groups in the pyramid (e.g. "Bread, Cereal, Rice, and Pasta Group"), the groups will be referred to in this book as "Grain Group," "Fruit Group," "Vegetable Group," "Dairy Group," and "Protein Group."

CONCEPTS TO TEACH The following points outline the key messages children should grasp when studying the Food Guide Pyramid.

• Why a pyramid shape? Using a 3-dimensional pyramid model (available in many math kits), explain how the pyramid is wide at the bottom and very narrow at the top. The Food Guide Pyramid (refer to poster) relies on a base of grains, which provide the foundation of our diet. A strong pyramid also needs plenty of fruits and vegetables, dairy and protein foods, but only a small amount of fatty and sugary foods.

To demonstrate, ask a child to balance the pyramid model on its base (easy!). Next, ask if anyone would like to try to balance it on its tip (impossible!). In the same way, a diet of mostly greasy, sugar-laden "tip foods" cannot possibly be balanced.

• Each group provides certain "nutrients" that help our body work at its best. The body needs a total of about 40 nutrients which fall into six general classes: **Carbohydrates**, **Protein**, **Fat**, **Vitamins**, **Minerals**, and **Water**. Eating foods from all the food groups is one way to get the nutrients needed for good health (See Table 4-3 on page 36).

• We need the most servings of grains (6-11 each day) because they are rich in energy-giving carbohydrates and fiber. Our body's first and most important need is for energy. Besides the energy it takes for play and sports, we also use energy

TABLE 4-3

NUTRIENTS AND THEIR WORK

FOOD GROUP	KEY NUTRIENTS*	ACTION IN THE BODY
Grains	Carbohydrate, fiber, B vitamins, iron	**Carbohydrate** is the body's major source of energy. **B vitamins** help in the body's use of energy. **Fiber** aids the movement of food through the digestive tract. **Iron** carries oxygen in red blood cells and muscle cells.
Vegetables	Vitamin A, Vitamin C, Folic Acid, Iron, Magnesium, Fiber	**Vitamin A** helps maintain skin and mucous membranes and aids in vision. **Vitamin C** helps the body heal and fight infections. **Folic acid** is needed for healthy blood cells and is important for cell division, such as in pregnancy and growth. **Magnesium** is found in bones and is important for muscle and nerve functioning.
Fruits	Vitamin A, Vitamin C, Potassium, Folic Acid, Fiber	**Potassium** maintains the heart beat, regulates body fluids, and is needed for muscle and nerve functioning.
Protein	Protein, B vitamins, Iron, Zinc	**Protein** provides the building blocks needed for growth, replacement, and maintenance of body tissues. **Zinc** is necessary for healing, taste perception, growth, and sexual development.
Dairy	Calcium, Riboflavin, Protein	**Calcium** is needed for the development and maintenance of healthy bones and teeth. **Riboflavin** is a B vitamin that helps the body use energy.
"Use Sparingly" (Not a food group)	(Simple) Carbohydrates, Fat	**Simple carbohydrates** or sugars provide energy but few other nutrients. **Fat** is a source of energy and helps in the absorption of certain vitamins.

There are more than 40 different nutrients with many different functions that are required for good health. Each food group contributes many other nutrients in addition to the "key nutrients," listed here.

just to keep us alive. With each breath, heartbeat, or blink of the eyes, we are "spending" energy.

Fiber, while not exactly a nutrient, helps the body to move food through our systems. Fiber also helps our health in other ways, too (i.e. some fibers lower blood cholesterol and stabilize blood sugar levels). Whole grains such as brown rice and 100% whole wheat bread have more fiber than refined white rice or bread made from enriched flour. (Other fiber-rich foods include beans, fruits, and vegetables.)

• The fruit and vegetable groups are important because they give us many vitamins, minerals, carbohydrates, and fiber. We need at least 2 servings of fruit and 3 servings of vegetables each day for good health and good looks, too! The vitamins and minerals in fruits and vegetables help keep our skin, eyes, and hair looking healthy.

• While protein and dairy group foods are vital for good health, fewer servings are recommended. Dairy foods give our bodies protein, calcium, and riboflavin while the protein group is rich in protein, iron, and zinc. Most children need two daily servings (or a total of 5-7 ounces) of protein foods. Since youth is an important bone-building time, three servings of dairy products are recommended for children each day. To lower fat intake, choose **lean** meats, chicken without the skin, fish, beans, and **lowfat** dairy foods.

• How do you know the right number of servings for you? The servings listed in the Food Guide Pyramid give ranges, like 2-4, or 6-11.

Most children need to eat at least the minimum number of servings for proper nutrition. But many kids will need more, especially those who are active in sports and play. The best way to know how much to eat is to listen to your body! Eat until your body feels full ... but not too full. You should feel satisfied but not overly stuffed. (This is a good place for a discussion on how it feels to eat too much, not enough, and just the right amount).

• Examples of foods classified in the tip of the pyramid include soda pop, candy, margarine, butter, and oil. These foods are not poisonous or terrible. Even the most well-planned, healthful diet includes some fats and sugars. But just as the tip of the pyramid is a small piece of the whole, "tip" foods are a small piece of a healthful diet.

Foods high in fat and sugar are low in nutrients and, in excess, contribute to health problems such as heart disease, obesity, and cancer. Eating too many greasy, sugary foods can also leave us feeling sluggish instead of energized.

Some foods in the main five food groups contain fat and sugar, too. The symbols splashed throughout the pyramid illustrate the relative levels of fat and sugar in all food groups. They remind us, for instance, that some fruits are canned in heavy sweetened syrup or potatoes processed into french fries are high in fat. A limitation of the pyramid is the failure to rank the fat content of foods within groups (i.e. beans as opposed to sausage or cheese compared to nonfat yogurt). Careful label reading can help children to distinguish between high and low fat foods within each group (See Chapter 6).

AVOIDING "PYRAMID OVERLOAD" Break pyramid concepts into several sessions so children can fully "digest" the material. Each session should ideally have a hands-on, discovery activity (See next section for ideas). Below is a suggested timeline for presenting information, although it will vary according to age and developmental level:

Session 1—Introduce the Food Guide Pyramid poster, discuss the shape using a 3-D model, and explain how foods for good health are divided into five main food groups. Plan activities that allow students to sort and categorize foods into the five food groups.

Session 2—Review the number of servings suggested from each food group. (see Table 4-2). Lead the class in a discussion of "How many servings do I need?" Set up measuring centers where students can discover the serving sizes of various foods.

Session 3—Introduce the concept of nutrients and list the six classes (Carbohydrates, Protein, Fat, Vitamins, Minerals, Water). Explain that because each food group contains a different set of nutrients, we need foods from all the groups to get the nutrients our body needs. Highlight how key nutrients are needed to build and maintain a healthy body (See Table 4-3).

Session 4—Ask the class for examples of foods that fit into the tip of the pyramid. Discuss the concept of dietary excess, i.e. how we need to limit foods which are high in sugar and fat. Point out the symbols (small circles and triangles) used throughout the pyramid that show relative fat and sugar content of different foods.

Planning Pyramid Activities

To bring alive the concepts of the pyramid, plan activities that will engage students and make the pyramid relevant to their lives.

ACTIVITIES

13 USES FOR A BLANK PYRAMID The blank pyramids on pages 40 and 41 can be used in a variety of ways to teach pyramid concepts. Photocopy, enlarge, or redraw for use with students. Assign children the following activities or create your own.

1. Trace the pyramid onto paper plates. Draw a picture of each food and drink you had for breakfast in the correct place on the pyramid. Do the same for lunch, dinner, or snacks. Is your pyramid plate balanced? Does each meal include at least three of the five food groups? Do snacks have at least two of the food groups?

2. Use the lined pyramid as a daily diet record. Carry it with you and record each food you eat or drink in the appropriate food group space. Break foods into their components, e.g. record a soup made of noodles, beef, and vegetables in the grains, protein, and vegetable groups. Check your record for balance. Is there lots of blank space in certain groups? Are other groups overcrowded? Are there changes you could make to better balance your "personal pyramid?"

3. Chart today's school breakfast or lunch menu on the pyramid. Are the menus balanced? Would you make any changes in the meals?

4. Ask the children who brought a packed lunch from home to analyze the contents and record on the pyramid. Are most of the food groups represented? Would you make any changes in the meal?

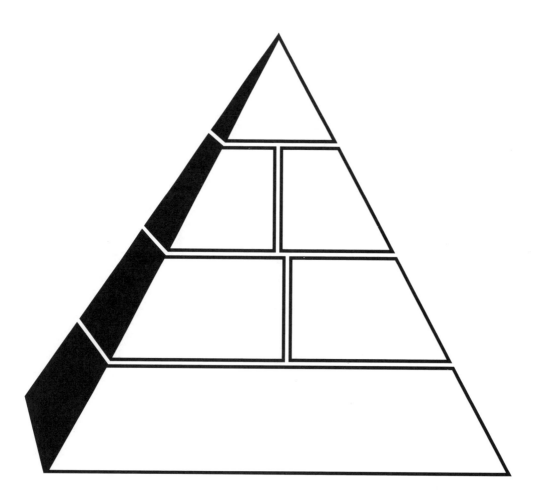

Enlarge and reproduce for educational use.

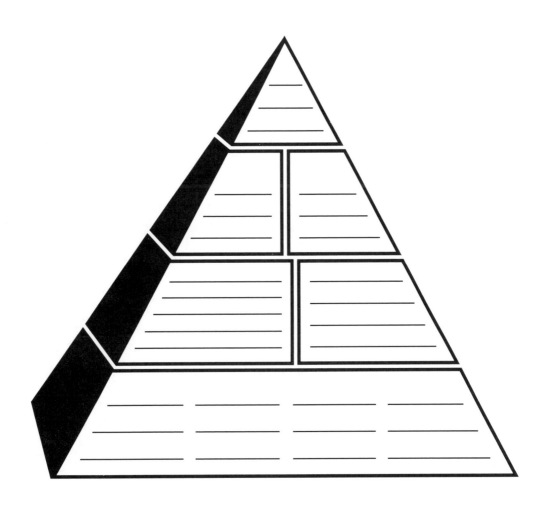

Enlarge and reproduce for educational use.

5. Use the pyramid to plan your after-school or bedtime snack. Close your eyes and think about the foods that are usually available in your refrigerator or cupboard. Next, think about which of these foods would make a good "pyramid snack." Write down or draw this snack on your pyramid. Be sure to include foods that you like to eat!

6. Plan a pyramid meal that you can cook yourself. It can be as simple as a peanut butter/fruit sandwich with milk or as complicated as a spaghetti dinner with salad. You're the cook!

7. Draw a vegetarian pyramid. What foods would you include in the protein group? What about the dairy group? Do vegetarians eat eggs? (ANSWER: Vegetarian diets are varied. Some, called lacto-vegetarians, include milk, yogurt, and cheese in their diets. Lacto-ovo-vegetarians also eat eggs. Strict vegetarians, known as vegans, eat only plant-based foods and often include calcium-fortified soy milk and tofu in their diets.)

8. Draw an ethnic pyramid. Pick a culture that you are studying about or interested in and research what types of foods they commonly eat. For example, a Mexican pyramid might include tortillas (grains), beans (protein), cheese (dairy), and salsa (vegetables). What would a Middle Eastern, Chinese, or Italian pyramid look like?

9. Using the lined pyramid, dissect combination foods and write the components on the pyramid. Use one of the following examples or create your own:

> VEGETARIAN PIZZA: whole wheat crust, tomato sauce with spices, part-skim mozzarella cheese, red pepper rings, mushrooms, onions, black olives
>
> CHINESE STIR-FRY: water chestnuts, bean sprouts, pea pods, broccoli florets, chicken pieces, peanuts, rice
>
> SUB SANDWICH: Whole Wheat french roll, sliced turkey, lean ham, part-skim mozzarella cheese, tomato slices, shredded lettuce, alfalfa sprouts, oil, vinegar

10. Research the nutrients that each food group provides. Write the key nutrients from each group on the lined pyramid. (ANSWERS: Grains—carbohydrate, fiber, B vitamins, iron; Vegetables—vitamins A and C, folic acid, fiber, iron, magnesium; Fruits—vitamins A and C, folic acid, potassium, fiber; Dairy—calcium, protein, riboflavin; Protein—protein, iron, zinc, B vitamins; Refer to Table 4-3 for more about specific nutrients).

11. Draw a "body-part" pyramid that represents how each food group helps the body. EXAMPLE: Draw an exercising body in the grain space, healthy eyes in the vegetable group, glowing hair and skin for the fruit group, an arm posing a muscle in the protein group, and a healthy, toothy smile for the dairy group.

12. Make a giant pyramid to decorate the school cafeteria. Start with a large blank pyramid. Assign eleven students to the grain group, five to the vegetable group, four to the fruit group, three to the milk group, three to the protein group, and two to the fats, oil, and sweets category (you may need to make adjustments according to class size). Have students design, draw, paint or color a favorite food from their assigned food group. Paste them on the large food pyramid and hang in the cafeteria. Be sure to have students sign their artwork.

Or, with the help of an artist or art teacher, have students design and paint a pyramid mural right on the cafeteria wall!

13. HOMEWORK: Accompany the "family shopper" on the next trip to the grocery store. Are most foods in the store from one of the five food groups? Is your family shopping cart heavy on grains, fruits, and vegetables, with medium amounts of dairy and protein foods, and just a few fats and sweets? As the groceries are being put away at home, write down all the items on your lined pyramid. Is your pyramid balanced? What suggestions would you give the family shopper (nicely, of course!)?

MAKE A PYRAMID COUNTER Using a shoebox, string or twine, and buttons or beads, children can make a device to help them count how many food group servings they eat each day. First, punch six small holes along one of the long sides of the shoe box. Punch six more on the other side that pair up with the first set of holes. Next, cut six pieces of string that are approximately twice the width of the box. Knot each piece of string and thread through the holes. Feed 12 beads or buttons onto each string. The last step is to thread the string through the opposite hole, and tie a knot on the end to secure.

Each row of beads represents a food group. To match the *Food Guide Pyramid*, order the groups so that the grain group is on the bottom, followed by vegetables, fruits, dairy, protein, and the "tip" on the top. (Children may want to write the food groups on the bottom of the box before stringing beads.)

Ask students to write down the foods they eat each day (The pyramid diet record suggested in #2 above works well). Using the "pyramid counter," the students can move one bead to the opposite side for each serving they eat in that category. They can also do this for individual meals, snacks, or school meal menus. This device will give students a visual tool that allows them to immediately gauge whether a meal or diet is "pyramid shaped."

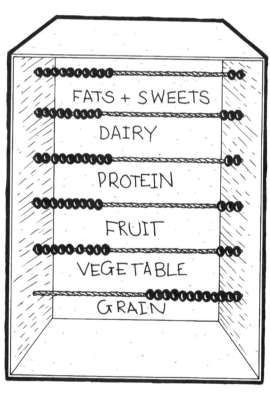

⊞ MEASURING CENTERS

Perhaps the biggest hangup in applying the *Food Guide Pyramid* to daily eating habits is confusion over serving sizes (this is true of adults as well as children). Hands-on experience weighing and measuring different foods will give children a better grasp of what a "serving" really means.

Set up centers for children to manipulate and measure real food. Small food scales, measuring cups, measuring spoons, plates, cups, and bowls are needed for this activity.

CAUTION: This is NOT an eating activity since everyone will be touching the food. You may want to plan this activity in conjunction with a snack or conduct it right after lunch, when tummies are full!.

Some suggestions for centers:

• Measure one serving (1/2 cup) of cooked spaghetti, noodles, macaroni, or rice onto a "dinner-sized" plate.

• Weigh two ounces of cheese in different forms, including sliced, cubed, or grated. (1 1/2–2 ounces is considered a serving).

• Measure 1 teaspoon of soft margarine or slice 1 "pat" of cubed butter (using lines on butter wrapper).

• Pour 6 ounces (3/4 cup) of unsweetened fruit juice into a glass.

• Using whole leaves from leaf lettuce or fresh spinach, tear into bite-sized pieces and measure 1 cup. How many lettuce leaves does it take to make one serving?

• Weigh 2 ounces of canned tunafish.

• Set up a "guess table" with a variety of foods. The objective is to guess how many servings each food item really provides. Examples include an english muffin (2 servings), 1 cup canned fruit (2 servings), 1 medium orange (1 serving), 1 cup cooked oatmeal (2 servings), 1/2 pint carton of milk (1 serving), or a 3 ounce cooked hamburger patty (1 serving).

Your school cafeteria manager is the real expert when it comes to serving sizes. Part of the manager's job is to serve the right-sized portions. Invite him/her into the classroom to demonstrate different scoops, scales, and spoons used to control serving sizes. Also encourage students to take note of the serving sizes on their school breakfast and lunch tray. For instance, each school lunch has 2 ounces meat or protein, 1 cup milk, 1-2 servings of grains, and (usually) 1 fruit serving and 1 vegetable serving.

USING THE PYRAMID IN DRAMATIC PLAY AREAS Setting up dramatic play areas is a great way for primary students (grades K-2) to play and practice the concepts of the *Food Guide Pyramid*.

Pyramid Supermarket: Set up a supermarket that is full of pyramid choices. Include shelves for food, grocery carts, aprons, cash register, and grocery bags. Decorate the walls with student-made posters and advertisements.

> **YOU WILL NEED:**
> - Shelves
> - A variety of empty food packages and/or food models
> - Grocery carts
> - Aprons
> - Cash register
> - Grocery sacks

For food models, use empty food packages (stuff items such as bread bags and flour sacks with pillow foam), canned goods, milk cartons, packages of rice, beans, and pasta, and plastic or rubber models of perishable items such as fruits, vegetables, meats, and eggs. Include a wide variety of foods from all five food groups and a few foods from the pyramid tip.

Pyramid Kitchen: Stock the dramatic play area kitchen with healthful pyramid choices. Include models of low or nonfat milk, yogurt, and cheese, lean meats, chicken, and fish, whole grains, including 100% whole wheat bread and flour, and plenty of grains, beans, fruits and vegetables.

The Pyramid Cafe: Use glasses, plates, silverware, napkins and food pictures that students can make into meals. The food pictures can be pre-printed, cut from magazines, or made by students. (The food model pictures available from National Dairy Council are especially good because they represent actual-size servings—see Appendix B.)

> **YOU WILL NEED:**
> - Durable glasses, plates, silverware and napkins
> - Tables and chairs
> - Food models or sturdy food pictures
> - Aprons
> - Chef hats
> - Cash register
> - Pads and pencils
> - Menus (made by students)

Provide tables and chairs, student-created menus, aprons, chef hats, pads and pencils, a cash register, and anything else your young restaurateurs need to run their cafe.

A PYRAMID PARTY: CREATE YOUR OWN SANDWICH A great cooking/tasting activity is to create pyramid sandwiches. Check with your cafeteria manager as a source for low-cost food supplies. If eaten as part of a reimbursable school meal, the food items will count as meal components. Funds for nutrition education projects may also be available from the local parent-teacher organization or through nutrition education grants (See Appendix B).

NOTE: It is best to conduct this activity as part of lunch or at the end of the school day to avoid interfering with the school meal program.

> **YOU WILL NEED:**
> - Plenty of volunteers!
> - Variety of food items from each food group (see text for examples)
> - Serving utensils
> - Long table
> - Plastic or latex gloves
> - Plates
> - Plastic knives
> - Napkins

Review Appendix A, "Guidelines for Safe Classrooom Cooking," before setting up this activity. Be sure to enlist parent volunteers to help with this project.

To create pyramid sandwiches, make available a variety of items that can be combined in an infinite number of sandwich combinations. Try to have at least three choices from each food group available. Below are examples from each food category.

Grains: whole wheat bread, rye bread, bagel, tortilla, English muffin, pita bread, French rolls

Vegetables: lettuce or spinach leaves, tomato slices, cucumber slices, pepper rings, alfalfa sprouts, onion slices, mushroom slices

Fruits: banana slices, raisins, applesauce, pineapple tidbits, blueberries, kiwi slices

Dairy: lowfat ricotta cheese, lowfat cheese slices, lowfat grated cheese, nonfat plain and fruit flavored yogurt

<u>Protein:</u> peanut butter, lean sliced turkey, ham, or roastbeef, water-packed tuna, refried beans

<u>Fats & Sweets:</u> butter, margarine, mayonnaise, jam, jelly

Before you start, list all the available food items on the board. Explain that students will get a chance to build their own pyramid sandwich, using any combination of foods they wish. Encourage them to start thinking about the sandwich they wish to make—otherwise the line may move at a snails pace! (An amusing book to read ahead of time is *"What's Cooking, Jenny Archer?"* by Ellen Conford—see page 58 for a detailed description).

On a long table, set out items, grouped by food group. You will also need plastic gloves, plates, plastic knives for spreading, and napkins. After thorough handwashing, let small groups of children come to the table. Instruct them to put on plastic gloves and refrain from touching their hair, face, clothing, or neighbor.

Encourage students to experiment with new food combinations, building a sandwich which has at least three of the five food groups. After everyone has created a pyramid sandwich, it's time to eat the results!

Follow-up Activities Encourage students to write about their sandwich, including what they liked about it, how they would change it next time, how many servings of each food group they used, and whether they think their family or friends would eat it.

The food lists on the board can also be used:

• To create additional sandwich combinations on paper that the children could try at home.

• To construct sentences or a story, using as many of the food words as possible.

• As weekly spelling words.

CHAPTER 5

LANGUAGE ARTS

"Thank you for coming to our classroom and telling us about good food. I checked out this one book and it showed things like how to do a mouse out of a potato and this other stuff."–Brittany

Children can discover a variety of nutrition concepts through language arts. Nutrition can be effectively integrated into reading, writing, storytelling, and even spelling activities.

Daily Menu Reading

As you change the calendar and discuss the weather each day, consider another daily task—read and discuss the school lunch menu (and perhaps the following day's breakfast menu).

Assign a student to read the menu to the class. As time allows, ask students questions about the menu, such as:

• What food groups are represented in the menu? Does it fit the guidelines of the *Food Guide Pyramid*?

• Poll students to find out how many will eat the school meal. How many brought their lunch from home?

• Ask children what they like the most and least about the menu. Encourage them to fill in the blank, "If I were the cafeteria manager, I would serve_____."

• Predict how many students schoolwide will eat the school meal today. How can they find out the answer to their prediction? (HINT: Ask the cafeteria manager).

Children's Books With Food Themes

Children's literature is full of books with whimsical food themes. Many of the titles below will stimulate discussion, serve as a prelude to a nutrition or cooking activity, and promote positive food behavior.

EARLY ELEMENTARY (K-2ND GRADES)

Bread and Jam for Frances, by Russell Hoban, Scholastic Books, 1964. This book is a perfect antidote for children who make limited food choices. Frances' food jag is short-lived once her parents begin serving her bread and jam for every meal and snack. In the end, she agrees with her friend Albert, who declares, "I think it's nice that there are all different kinds of lunches and breakfasts and dinners and snacks. I think eating is nice."

ACTIVITY
- Lead a discussion on how choosing a variety of different foods can make eating fun. Encourage children to draw pictures of two or more different breakfasts, lunches, or dinners (with no repeating of foods) that they like to eat.

Blueberries for Sal, by Robert McCloskey, The Viking Press, 1948. Little Sal gets so involved picking (and eating) blueberries on Blueberry Hill that she loses her mother. Meanwhile, a baby bear cub does the same—and soon the baby bear and Little Sal have swapped moms!

ACTIVITIES
- Sample and rate a variety of berries, including blueberries, strawberries, raspberries, etc.
- Research or discuss how blueberries and other berries grow. In late Spring/early Summer, take a field trip to a berry farm.

YOU WILL NEED:
- Different berries for tasting
- Plastic gloves
- Serving bowls and utensils
- Small plates

Eating the Alphabet: Fruits & Vegetables From A to Z, by Lois Ehlert, Harcourt Brace Jovanovich, 1989. With beautiful watercolor illustrations, the art in this book will appeal to readers of all ages. The author includes well-known produce with the more exotic, including endive, jicama, kumquat, kohlrabi, quince, ugli fruit, and xigua (Chinese watermelon). A highlight of the book is the glossary, which gives descriptions, origins, and interesting facts about all of the fruits and vegetables in the book.

ACTIVITIES

• Bring in a variety of the fruits and vegetables from *Eating the Alphabet* to observe and taste.

• Take a walking fieldtrip to a grocery market. Tour the produce section, noting the variety of produce available. Write about it later.

Encourage students to create and illustrate their own "Eating the Alphabet" books, using foods from any group they wish.

Assign each student a letter of the alphabet. Distribute brown paper bags and assorted art supplies, instructing students to make a puppet which represents a food of that letter. Use the puppets to create a skit or act out "The Alphabet Song" (See Chapter 9 for more ideas).

YOU WILL NEED:
- A variety of fruits and vegetables
- Cutting board and knife
- Plastic gloves
- Serving bowls and utensils
- Small plates

YOU WILL NEED:
- Small paper lunch bags
- Art supplies

Eating Fractions, by Bruce McMillan, Scholastic Inc., 1991. A math book that whets the appetite, the bright color photos in this book show two kids eating delicious "fractions" of food. A banana, cloverleaf roll, vegetable pizza, corn-on-the-cob, pear salad, and strawberry pie illustrate math concepts. The author carries his math (and food) message one step further by including his recipes, which provide delicious practice learning fractions.

ACTIVITIES

• Use a cantaloupe or honeydew melon to illustrate fractions and provide a healthy snack. In a stepwise fashion, cut the melon in half, fourths, eighths, etc. depending on the size of the melon. Pass out for snack, asking students what "fraction" of the whole they are eating.

YOU WILL NEED:
- Melons
- Cutting board and knife
- Plastic gloves
- Small plates or napkins

• For homework, ask students to find and report on a "fraction" of a food they ate at home, e.g. 1/8 of a pizza, 1/12 of a casserole, or 1/2 of an apple.

Fat, Fat Rose Marie, by Lisa Passen, Henry Holt, 1991. The new girl at school, Rose Marie endures cruel teasing by all of her classmates except Claire. Freckle-faced Claire notices Rose Marie's shiny blond hair, bright blue eyes, and talent for math. Individual acceptance and the true meaning of friendship are themes explored in this book.

ACTIVITIES

• Lead a discussion on how people come in a variety of shapes, colors, and sizes, pointing out that there is no one "best" way to look. Discuss the concept of prejudice and elicit ways that children can deal with mean teasing and cruel remarks.

Have students create life-sized self portraits, tracing their bodies onto large sheets of paper. Have them draw and color in the details, emphasizing their own unique qualities. Display in the classroom or hallway.

Gobble and Gulp, by Stephen Cosgrove, Random House, 1985. One in a series of stories about the Whimsies, "Gobble and Gulp" tells of how the Whimsies loved to grow and eat wholesome foods. But trouble brews for Whimsie twins Blossom and Sprout when they are placed under a spell from Switch Witch. They ignore the foods that are good for them and stuff themselves with sweets. The spell is broken when they discard the "Sweet Tooth" necklaces given to them by Switch Witch.

ACTIVITIES

• This book reinforces the role excessive sugar plays in tooth decay. Lead a discussion on how bacteria in the mouth love sugar too! When the bacteria feed on sugars, acid is formed which can harm teeth and result in cavities.

Conduct an experiment with soda pop and a tooth (ask your dentist for donations or use a baby tooth). Place the tooth in the soda pop and observe and

YOU WILL NEED:
- Tooth
- Soda pop
- Latex gloves

record changes each day. The acid and sugar from the pop will eventually dissolve the tooth!

NOTE: When handling teeth, be sure to wear latex gloves to minimize the risk of disease transmission.

Green Eggs and Ham, by Dr. Seuss, Random House, 1960.
Tongue-tied teachers and parents can take refuge in the fact that "Green Eggs and Ham" does make an important point about food—you will never know if you like a new food until you try it. That now classic refrain is as pertinent today as ever: "You do not like them. So you say. Try them! Try them! And you may. Try them and you may, I say."

ACTIVITY
• Have children think of foods that they are hesitant to try, either at home or at school. Award "Sam-I-Am" points each time a child tries any new food of their choice. Reward students with small incentives or privileges after they attain a certain number of points.

Mrs. Pig's Bulk Buy, by Mary Rayner, Atheneum, 1981. This book provides yet another twist on the theme that variety is essential when making food choices. Mrs. Pig teaches her ten piglets a lesson when they insist on dumping ketchup on everything, even toast, salad, and eggs! On her next trip to the store, she buys six enormous jars of ketchup. At first, the piglets are excited that they get so much of their favorite food. But once they realize that's all they get, they soon crave real food. The fanciful illustrations in this book show the little pigs gradually changing from white to pink.

ACTIVITY
• Set up the following scenario for children: If you could eat only one food, what would it be? How soon would you get tired of this food? Write a make-believe story of what might happen if you ate too much of this one food.

Stone Soup, by Marcia Brown, Charles Scribner's Sons, 1947.
A classic story of how three hungry soldiers convince the peasants of a small village that soup made of stones is indeed hearty and delicious. As the soldiers

begin heating up their soup of water and three polished stones, the peasants eagerly contribute ingredients, including a few carrots, some cabbage, a little barley, beef, potatoes, and milk, until finally the soldiers declare the soup "fit for a King."

ACTIVITY

- As a class, create a pot of vegetable-stone soup, using a crock pot and clean stone. Use tomato or vegetable juice for the base, add salt, pepper, and desired seasonings, and ask each child to bring a fresh vegetable from home. Assemble first thing in the morning, cook on high, and eat for a snack during the later part of the school day!

YOU WILL NEED:
- Crock pot
- Clean stone
- Tomato or vegetable juice
- Salt, pepper, seasonings
- Assorted vegetables (from children)
- Soup ladle
- Bowls and spoons

The Berenstain Bears and Too Much Junk Food, by Stan and Jan Berenstain, Random House, 1985. When Mama Bear notices her two cubs getting a little chubby, she decides to curtail their junk-food habits. To his surprise, Papa Bear must forgo much of his junk food as well. Great family reading, the Berenstains do an excellent job of covering basic nutrition principles, the importance of a healthy lifestyle, and the role exercise plays in good health.

ACTIVITIES

- Ask children to write down or draw physical activities that their family can do together.

Lead a discussion on how exercise and nutrition work together to produce fit young bodies.

The Little Red Hen (Authors, publishers, and versions vary slightly—I prefer the version where she makes bread, not cake). While this classic sends a strong message about work, cooperation, and consequences, an underlying theme teaches children the stages of bread production. From wheat seed to bread, the Little Red Hen perseveres in her production of a loaf of bread.

ACTIVITIES

Use visual props and a baking activity to tell the story. Obtain wheat kernels (purchase from mills or specialty grocery stores), stalks of dried wheat (available in craft stores), whole wheat flour, and whole wheat bread dough (from scratch or purchased frozen). After the story, divide the bread dough into roll-sized portions for each student. Encourage children to create their own "bread art" by kneading and shaping the dough. Line baking tray with parchment baking paper, label each child's bread art, bake according to package or recipe instructions, and serve as a snack. (You may want to enlist the help of your cafeteria manager with this project.)

Using potting soil and small containers (empty milk cartons work great), have students plant the wheat kernels and care for their plants (See Chapter 7 for more on growing plants).

The Milkmakers, by Gail Gibbons, MacMillan Inc., 1985.
Full of bright, colorful illustrations, this book explains in detail how a dairy cow generates milk and how the milk is processed prior to its eventual arrival at the table.

ACTIVITY
• Take a field trip to a dairy or dairy farm.

The Very Hungry Caterpillar, by Eric Carle, Philomel Books, 1983. This story clearly and vividly illustrates how food is needed to build young bodies. The caterpillar, with his insatiable appetite, eventually grows big and prepares to turn into a beautiful butterfly. This book sets the stage for a discussion of how food fuels the growth of all living things, even kids.

ACTIVITIES

• Encourage children to create a story about "The Very Hungry Kid," complete with the foods they (or the character they create) would choose to eat on each day of the week and the resultant growth that occurs.

To measure how food fuels the growth of children, start a classroom growth chart. Take measurements each month, noting the changes as the year progresses.

When I'm Hungry, by Jane R. Howard, Dutton, 1992. Imagine eating bananas right off the tree like a monkey or lapping milk from a bowl puppy-style. As the boy in this story munches his breakfast, he imagines eating like different animals do. In the end, he decides it's best to eat from a plate and drink from a glass "right in the middle of my very own family."

ACTIVITIES

• Ask the children which animal they would prefer to be and why. Suggest they write or draw about the eating habits of this animal.

• Just as animals have different ways of eating, people also have different eating habits and traditions. Ask the students to describe a meal with friends or family that has been especially memorable (See Chapter 8 for more on identifying family food customs).

UPPER ELEMENTARY (3RD-5TH GRADES)

Annie Pitts, Artichoke, by Diane deGroat, Simon & Schuster, 1992. Third-grader Annie Pitts is determined to become a famous actress. But she fails to get the lead in the class nutrition play after a food fight with Matthew at the supermarket fieldtrip. Forced to play the artichoke (and a last minute fill-in for the fish), Annie manages to put on a performance that nobody will forget! Students will enjoy this humorous book as they learn a few nutrition concepts, too.

ACTIVITY

As a class or in small groups, stage a nutrition play. See Chapter 9 for ideas.

Benjy and the Power of ZINGIES, by Jean Van Leeuwen, Dial, 1982.
Third grader Benjy is small for his age and frustrated by his attempts to match
the athletic skill of the boys who tease and taunt him. He sets out to "build a
better body" by eating "Zingies," a breakfast cereal touted by the fictional
superstar athlete Clyde Johnson. Convinced that Zingies "build better bodies
eight ways," Benjy eats them for breakfast, snacks, on his sandwiches, etc.
Unable to budge the scale even one pound, Benjy ultimately realizes that size
is more a matter of genetics than Zingies.

ACTIVITY
- Discuss the motives behind food advertising. Ask students if ads for food
products are always true. (See page 110 for more activity ideas that explore
food advertising.)

***FOODWORKS—Over 100 Science Activities and Fascinating Facts that
Explore the Magic of Food***, by the Ontario Science Centre, Addison-Wesley, 1987.
This book will interest children and adults alike with its amazing collection of food
experiments, food facts, and games, all with an emphasis on health. This book
answers off-beat food questions such as why there's no such thing as Chinese
cheese, why people in hot climates eat spicy-hot food, who invented noodles, what
the worlds' largest crop is, or why potatoes were once illegal in France.

Nutrition, What's in the Food We Eat, by Dorothy Hinshaw Patent, Holiday
House, 1992. A very straightforward book with wonderful color photographs, the
author explains the basics of nutrition in a very clear, direct style. Explanations
of how the body uses food, the six classes of nutrients, advice for healthy eating, and a glossary of terms are covered in this book, making it a good reference for students involved in nutrition projects or reports.

Nothing's Fair in Fifth Grade, by Barthe DeClements, Viking Penguin, 1981.
Written by a school counselor, this fictional story explores the psychological
issues surrounding childhood obesity. Not only is Elsie Edwards the new girl at
school, she is also obese and considered "gross" by classmates. Elsie's classmates

eventually accept her and she begins to lose weight. This book teaches valuable lessons about the prejudice and cruelty endured by fat people in our society.

ACTIVITY

• Lead a discussion on how people come in a variety of shapes and sizes, pointing out that there is no one "best" way to look.

What's Cooking, Jenny Archer?, by Ellen Conford, Little, Brown, and Co., 1989. A "creative" cook who enjoys sandwiches made with mint jelly and bologna on raisin bread, Jenny begins concocting her own lunches for school. Soon her friends want her to make their lunches too. Figuring she will quickly get rich, Jenny sets out to sell creative lunches to her friends. Her plan backfires when she is unable to please the picky palates of her friends.

ACTIVITIES

• Create an original "pyramid sandwich." (See page 47).

Invite the school nutrition manager to class to discuss how he or she manages to meet the tastes and preferences of all the children in the school. Suggest that the class assist the manager in planning a school breakfast or lunch menu.

Putting A Nutrition Twist on Fairy Tales

A fun activity that sharpens writing, illustrating, storytelling, and comprehension skills is to retell classic stories, adding a nutritional bent. The possibilities for student assignments are endless—here are a few examples.

ACTIVITIES

• Remember Jack Sprat who ate no fat and his wife who ate no lean? What would you tell Jack and Mrs. Sprat about nutritional moderation?

• Write a letter to "Baby Bear," giving him ideas on added ingredients that would make his porridge extra delicious and nutritious.

• If Little Red Riding Hood was really concerned about her sick grandmother's health, what "goodies" should she pack in the basket that would help Granny stay healthy?

- Imagine that the witch in "Hansel and Gretel" was really a good witch, concerned with the nutritional health of the children who came to visit. Instead of gingerbread and candy, what foods would her house be made of?
- In the story of the grasshopper and the ant, the ant stocked up for the winter while the grasshopper failed to plan and went hungry. What advice would you give the grasshopper on collecting and storing food for the winter?
- The story of "Jack and the Beanstalk" fails to tell about the crop of beans that must have resulted from such a large plant. Write or tell about what Jack and his mom did with all those beans. Were they green beans or dried beans? Did they eat them or sell them? How did they cook them?
- When Winnie-the-Pooh indulges himself with too much honey and condensed milk at Rabbit's house, he gets stuck attempting to exit Rabbit's hole! How could Pooh Bear improve his diet so he doesn't get stuck the next time?

Descriptive Writing

Using food as a subject is an effective way to develop descriptive writing skills. While children may have limited experience in other areas, they encounter food several times each day. The novice writer can more easily describe scenes and objects that are based on first hand experience. Some ideas:

ACTIVITIES

- Food can evoke strong emotions—positive as well as negative. Suggest that students write about a particular meal or food that made them feel especially happy, excited, sad, grouchy, or even angry. Encourage them to provide details regarding the surroundings, people, food, and why they felt as they did.
- Bring in colorful pictures, posters, or samples of real food. Assign students the task of describing one food, using as many details as possible.
- Bring in various foods for a snack or tasting. Ask students to write down how different foods appeal to each of their five senses (e.g. The strawberry is a beautiful,

YOU WILL NEED:
- Colorful food pictures

OR

- A variety of real food samples to observe, smell, and taste red color with seeds that remind me of polka dots. When I bite into a carrot, the crunchy sound fills up my whole head. The smell of fresh bread makes me feel warm and happy clear down to my toes).

Writing Activities for the Young Nutrition Advocate

Starting at a young age, it is important that kids learn to voice their opinion about policies and messages that affect their nutrition choices. The goal of writing letters should be to communicate opinions in a clear, constructive manner. Two areas to target include school meals and food advertisements.

🍽 School Meals

ACTIVITIES

• Begin by writing letters to the school nutrition manager or district nutrition director. Suggest that children begin the letter by stating what they like best about the school meals. If there are comments, suggestions, or criticisms, word them in a constructive way, e.g. "One change I would like to see in the menu/cafeteria is_____" or "My idea of the perfect school breakfast/lunch menu is _____."

• Write to the United States Department of Agriculture (USDA), the federal agency that oversees child nutrition programs, including school breakfast and lunch. Again, tell them what you like the best about the school meal program and changes (if any) that you would like to see. Address your letters to: Department of Agriculture, Office of The Secretary, 14th and Independence Ave SW, Washington, DC 20250.

Food Advertisements

ACTIVITIES

• The next time you are watching television on Saturday morning, keep a list of the advertised foods that are low in nutrition such as candy, pop, or sugary cereal. Also keep a list of ads for healthful foods from the five food groups. Are there more ads for healthful foods or low-nutrition foods? (See worksheet on page 115.) You can write letters to those responsible for the ads, including the food company who advertises or the network itself.

To find the address for the food company, look at the food package the next time you go to the grocery store (or ask an adult to do it for you). Printed on the package is an address you can write to voice your opinion.

• Write to the television networks and let them know how you feel about their food advertising. The major networks can be reached at the following addresses:

- ◆ ABC/Capital Cities, 77 West 66th Street, New York, New York, 10023
- ◆ CBS, 51 West 52nd Street, New York, New York, 10019
- ◆ NBC, 30 Rockefeller Plaza, New York, New York, 10112
- ◆ Nickelodeon, 1515 Broadway, 20th Floor, New York, New York, 10036
- ◆ FOX Broadcasting, 10201 West Pico Boulevard, Los Angeles, CA, 90035

Spelling List

Include food and nutrition words in your list of weekly spelling words. Examples are listed below.

Food	Nutrition
Pyramid	Nutrient
Grain	Carbohydrate
Fruit	Protein
Vegetable	Fat
Dairy	Vitamin
Water	Mineral
Diet	Fiber
Healthy	Exercise

CHAPTER 6

MATH

"I liked it when you showed us how much fat and sugar were in those two lunches. I was surprised when you showed us how much fat was in the lunch with the Big Mac. I thought that was kind of gross."–**Dawn**

The subjects of Nutrition and Math are easily integrated and mutually beneficial. Whether counting daily servings from the food groups, calculating nutrients, or learning how to decipher the *Nutrition Facts* food label, the application of nutrition requires basic math skills. Likewise, math skills can be learned or reinforced through the use of real-life food activities by working with a recipe, dividing up portions, or making purchases at the food market.

One food-related math skill that comes naturally to children, even the very young, is division. Children think of it as "fair share," always mindful that they get their deserved allotment of animal crackers, grapes, or apple wedges. Build this natural inclination into a snacktime math lesson, using examples such as "There are 25 crackers left for table A—since there are five of you, how many do you each get?" Conversely, ask children how many graham crackers you need to buy if each student typically eats three squares.

Teaching Label Lessons

Label reading helps children sharpen their nutrition, math, and critical thinking skills. The following activities will help children interpret and apply the Nutrition Facts label information.

ACTIVITIES

WHAT'S YOUR SERVING SIZE? Serving sizes on food products are now more standard and realistic. Even so, the government view of a "serving" will not

TABLE 6-1

LEARNING TO USE THE NUTRITION FACTS FOOD LABEL

Officially in place since May of 1994, the new nutrition label makes it easy for kids to decipher the sugar content of fruit drinks or the fat rating of hot dogs. New labeling laws require a *Nutrition Facts* label on all packaged foods and fresh meats. Nutrition information is also available in the produce and seafood sections for the 20 most commonly eaten raw fruits/vegetables and seafood.

The revised food label sports several additions and deletions. In a nutshell, the highlights:

- Effort has been made to standardize serving sizes, bringing them in line with what people actually eat. There is also more consistency between similar products (e.g. most cold breakfast cereals list a one-cup serving).

- Gone are the exhaustive list of vitamins and minerals, replaced by four key nutrients of special concern to Americans, i.e. Vitamin A, Vitamin C, Calcium, and Iron (Manufacturers may include more nutrients on a voluntary basis).

- Welcome members to the new label lineup are values for sugar and dietary fiber. Once optional on the label, sugars, starches, and fiber were often lumped together under the carbohydrates heading. This information is especially handy when comparing the merits of kids' favorite breakfast cereals.

- While the new label stops short of reporting the percent of calories contributed by fat, that magic number is now within easy grasp (See Table 6-2 for calculation). Keep in mind, though, that the goal to slide under 30% calories from fat applies to the diet as a whole, not to individual foods. Even a high fat hunk of cheese can be tempered by pairing it with lowfat crackers and fruit wedges.

- Daily values (DV), the new label reference numbers, show the contribution that each targeted nutrient makes to the daily diet. Expressed as a percentage, the DV tells you whether a food is high or low in a nutrient like fat, sodium, cholesterol, or vitamin C. In general, a food with a %DV of 5% or less for a nutrient is considered low in that nutrient, a product is considered a "good source" of a nutrient if the %DV is between 10-19%, and "high" if the %DV is greater than 20%. Highly nutritious foods rank lower on the %DV for total fat, saturated fat, cholesterol, and sodium, and higher on the %DV for total carbohydrate, dietary fiber, vitamins and minerals.

- The new label features a standard chart that targets the daily recommended levels for fats, cholesterol, sodium, carbohydrate, and fiber at 2000 and 2500 calories. While a child's nutrient needs are highly individual, these reference values give a "ballpark" goal for daily intake. Estimated caloric needs of children range from 1800 for the average 4-6 year old to 2000 for a typical 7-10 year old.

- The labels now require more complete ingredient lists, even for those foods which use the government's "standard" recipes, such as mayonnaise, ketchup, or jelly. This change is especially important for those who have allergies or sensitivities to specific food additives.

Nutrition Facts

Serving Size ½ cup (114g)

Servings Per Container 4

Amount Per Serving

Calories 90   Calories from Fat 30

% **Daily Value***

Total Fat 3g	**5%**
Saturated Fat 0g	**0%**
Cholesterol 0mg	**0%**
Sodium 300mg	**13%**
Total Carbohydrate 13g	**4%**
Dietary Fiber 3g	**12%**
Sugars 3g	
Protein 3g	

Vitamin A	80%	•	Vitamin C	60%
Calcium	4%	•	Iron	4%

* Percent Daily Values are based on a 2,000 calorie diet. Your daily values may be higher or lower depending on your calorie needs:

	Calories	2,000	2,500
Total Fat	Less than	65g	80g
Sat Fat	Less than	20g	25g
Cholesterol	Less than	300mg	300mg
Sodium	Less than	2,400mg	2,400mg
Total Carbohydrate		300g	375g
Fiber		25g	30g

Calories per gram:

Fat 9   •   Carbohydrate 4   •   Protein 4

Source: Food & Drug Administration

always match individual needs or preferences. To make this point, bring in a large box of breakfast cereal, cereal bowls, and measuring cups. Cover or remove the *Nutrition Facts* label information from the box. Ask children, a few at a time, to pour themselves a "bowl of cereal," typical of

what they would eat for breakfast or a snack. Next, have students measure and record how much they poured into the bowl. After everyone has taken a turn, appoint one child to read aloud the serving amount listed on the label. Ask how many children measured the same amount, more, or less than the label serving size. Remind students that the nutrition information on the remainder of the label pertains to the standard label serving size. Ask what that means in different situations, i.e. "If a label lists 4 grams of dietary fiber and your serving size is half as much as the standard serving, how many grams of fiber did you eat?"

OPTIONAL: Make a class graph that visually shows individual differences in serving sizes. Have each student plot their serving amount on a poster-sized bar graph. Include a comparison bar that shows the serving size listed on the label.

CALORIES FROM FAT Calories in food come from either carbohydrate, protein, or fat. When gauging the nutritional merit of a food item, it is often helpful to look at the number of calories that come from fat. That is why "Calories from Fat" is listed next to "Calories" on the *Nutrition Facts* label.

Over the course of a day, the recommended goal is to eat a maximum of 30% of calories from fat. That does not mean every single food must fall below the 30% goal—higher fat foods can be balanced with lower fat foods to obtain a daily average of around 30%.

To obtain calories from fat in a given food, simply divide "Calories from Fat" by "Total Calories," and multiply by 100 for the percentage. This exercise is especially helpful when comparing two similar food items (See section below).

Using the *Nutrition Facts* label, encourage students to calculate the percentage of calories from fat in several food products.

NOTE: Since students don't always carry calculators, pencils, or paper, encourage the use of estimation in evaluating the nutrition content of foods.

For example, the estimated fat content of a package of cookies with 65 calories per serving and 35 calories from fat would be "almost one-half of the calories."

TABLE 6-2

HOW TO CALCULATE PERCENT CALORIES FROM FAT

To calculate percent calories from fat using the Nutrition Facts food label, simply divide CALORIES FROM FAT by TOTAL CALORIES and multiply times 100 to arrive at the percentage. The equation looks like this:

$$\frac{\text{Calories From Fat}}{\text{Total Calories}} \times 100 = \% \text{ Calories From Fat}$$

Example: A box of snack crackers provides 70 calories for a serving of 5 crackers. The "calories from fat" are listed as 20.

$$\frac{20}{70} \times 100 = 28.6\% \text{ Calories From Fat}$$

MAKING COMPARISONS The food label is a powerful tool for comparing similar food products. Younger children can begin by comparing one nutrient in different products, while students in the intermediate grades can learn to compare several parameters on a label. Suggest that students develop graphs or pictures with fractional pieces to illustrate the differences between foods.

Ten suggestions for comparing labels, ranked from simple to more complex, are listed below.

YOU WILL NEED:

• A variety of food labels

OR

• Observation and recording of label information during a fieldtrip to the grocery store

1. Sugar in Breakfast Cereal—Bring in a variety of cereal boxes. Locate "Sugars" on the label. On a piece of paper, rank the cereals in order of sugar content.

2. Total Fat in Crackers—Rank various crackers in order of "total fat" content.

3. Fat in Snack Foods—Compare the fat content in one serving of pretzels, chips, packaged popcorn, and snack crackers.

4. Fiber in Bread—Just because a bread is dark in color, it's not necessarily full of fiber. Compare the "Dietary Fiber" content of white bread, 100% whole wheat bread, and bread that is simply labeled "wheat."

5. Sugars in Unlikely Places—Various forms of sugar are commonly added to foods, even those we don't think of as "sweet." Send children on a "scavenger hunt" for foods which contain added sugars such as ketchup, spaghetti sauce, mayonnaise, baked beans, hot dogs, and certain breads.

6. Rating Lunch Meats—There is a notable difference in the fat, calorie, and sodium content of luncheon meats. For homework or as part of a class fieldtrip, assign students the task of finding and comparing at least five different lunch meats, e.g. lean ham or roast beef, different types of turkey meat, bologna, and salami. Note the difference in calories, fat, and sodium for a standard serving size. Which products are the best overall choice?

7. The Merits of Milk—"Two percent" milk sounds like it must be low in fat, but is it? Write down the Total Fat, Calories, and Calories from Fat for nonfat, 1%, 2%, and whole milk. Have students calculate the "percent calories from fat" in all four milks. Ask students why milk listed as 1% or 2% fat appears much higher in fat when using the "percent calories from fat" calculation. (Answer: 1% or 2% refers to fat by weight, which is low since most of the weight in milk comes from water.)

OPTIONAL: Compare the calcium content between different varieties of milk.

OPTIONAL: Compare the fat, sugar, and calorie content of various frozen desserts, including ice cream, ice milk, frozen yogurt, and sherbet.

8. Finding the "Better Butter"—Although spreads like butter, butter blends, and margarines are by nature mostly fat, the key nutritional difference is the amount of fat that is saturated. (Saturated fat is associated with higher blood cholesterol and an increased risk for heart disease in later life.)

Ask children to look at a variety of labels and rank them by the level of saturated fat. Note that there is a large difference in the saturated fat content of liquid, soft tub, and stick margarines. Students will discover that certain margarines have nearly as much saturated fat as butter!

Keep in mind, too, that the flavor of butter is preferred by many, especially chefs and those involved in fine food preparation. Their advice: Use real butter—just use less of it!

9. Noodle Know-How—Kids have gone noodle-crazy over oriental ramen noodles. They may be surprised to learn that many brands fare worse in fat and sodium content than an average serving of potato chips! Encourage students to read and evaluate their favorite ramen noodle label. Ask them to look for brands that are lower in fat during their next trip to the grocery store.

OPTIONAL: Ask students how the nutrition of ramen noodles compares to standard egg noodles.

10. Taking a Closer Look at Fruit(?) Snacks—If you believe the advertising and packaging, there are a whole array of processed "fruit snacks" just loaded with fruit. To dispel this myth, teach students how to read ingredient labels on packaged foods, pointing out that ingredients are listed from most to least, by weight. Ask them to read the ingredient labels on a variety of fruit snacks to see what order "fruit" or "fruit juice concentrate" falls in the ingredient list. Usually the "fruit" is listed third or fourth, behind various types of sugar, corn syrup, and gelatin.

Measuring Nutrients in Food

Children can best grasp the concept of "high fat" or "high sugar" when they can actually see the fat and sugar in a food. The activities below give students practice in weighing and measuring, provides reference for what a "gram" is, and visually displays the fat and sugar content of various foods.

ACTIVITIES

WHAT'S A GRAM? Nutrient information on food labels, recipes, restaurant brochures, and reference tables is mostly metric, with food components measured in grams and milligrams (1/1000 of a gram). Some nutrients, like vitamin D and iodine, are needed in such small amounts that they are measured in micrograms (one millionth of a gram!).

The weight of a gram is approximately that of a small paper clip. Using a gram scale, ask students to weigh different common items, including a paper clip, pencil, eraser, chalk, etc.

> **YOU WILL NEED:**
> - Gram scale
> - Paper clip and other common items
> - Soda pop label
> - Coffee filters
> - Sugar

Next, explain how the weight of many of the nutrients in food is also listed in grams. The average 12 ounce can of soda pop, for instance, contains about 40 grams of sugar. To demonstrate, first place a coffee filter on top of the scale. Next, show the students how to "zero" the scale. Fill the coffee filter until the scale registers 40 grams—resulting in a small mountain of sugar!

SETTING UP A CENTER To set up a center for students to weigh and measure the fat and sugar in foods, you will need a gram scale, teaspoons, one pound of sugar, one pound of vegetable shortening, coffee filters, small plastic plates, and food packages or labels.

> **YOU WILL NEED:**
> + Gram scale
> + Teaspoons
> + One pound of sugar
> + One pound of vegetable shortening
> + Coffee filters
> + Small plastic plates
> + Food packages or labels

Another way to measure grams is to use a teaspoon. A teaspoon of sugar or fat weighs approximately 4 grams, so students can measure the teaspoons of fat and sugar in food by dividing total grams by 4.

On a long table, set out a variety of food packages or labels. Examples include candy bars, granola bars, yogurt containers, cereal boxes, potato chips, pretzels, crackers, cookies, or fast food containers (nutrient analysis, including fat and sugar content, is usually available in the restaurant or upon request).

A few at a time, students will read the labels and measure the fat and sugar content of the different food items, using coffee filters for sugar and plastic plates for fat. Have them place the containers with fat and sugar in front of each food package or label until they have measured all foods. When they are done, instruct them to scoop the fat and sugar back into the original containers and allow another group of students to work the center. (NOTE: Plastic plates can be washed and reused many times.)

OPTIONAL: Consider a semi-permanent display of the fat and sugar in foods for the classroom or cafeteria. Invite other classes to observe and comment.

OPTIONAL: Using food labels, measure the fiber content (in grams) in a variety of breads and cereals, using bran cereal to represent fiber.

Graphing

A visual way to present and evaluate information is through the use of graphing. Nutrition goals, trends, and concepts become more meaningful when children can see them plotted on a graph. Graph paper, colored pencils or markers, and a ruler are all that is needed to complete the following bar or line graphs.

ACTIVITIES

• Using a completed one-day food record, explain how to count servings and graph daily food intake. After counting the number of servings from each of the five food groups and "tip" of the pyramid, students can compare foods eaten to the recommended servings in the *Food Guide Pyramid*. Ask them to explain what the graph shows about their diet. Based on the results, suggest they set personal nutrition goals.

• Have students graph personal nutrition or fitness goals. Examples include eating three servings of vegetables each day, limiting candy to one serving a day, or bike riding at least 20 minutes daily. The vertical axis should include numbers from 0 to 10 (for number of servings) or 0 to 60 minutes (for minutes spent bicycling). Place a red dot or line at the level which is the goal (if a bar

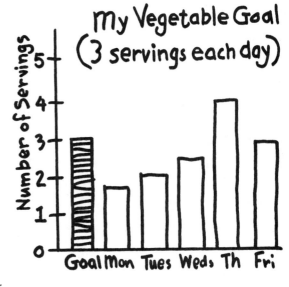

graph, draw a red bar which represents the goal). Underneath it, mark "G" for goal. Along the horizontal axis, write the days of the week.

Each day, keep track of how many servings or minutes. Plot results on the graph above the appropriate date. For line graphs, connect the dots to make a line. Ask students to explain their graph and report progress in meeting their goal.

• Pick one food group and survey the class to find out how many servings from that food group they ate yesterday. Assign groups of students to graph the data in various ways. For example, ask how many servings of fruit were consumed. On the board, write down the number of servings eaten by each student. Ask one group to compare the number of servings eaten by girls compared to boys. Another group can compare fruit intake between students who ate the school meal versus those who brought a lunch from home. Still another can compare fruit servings by table or group. Other ideas include comparing students by birthday month, eye or hair color, or whether their last name begins with a letter in the first or last half of the alphabet. (This activity is also a great way to reinforce skills in averaging numbers.)

Ask students to draw conclusions about the factors that might influence fruit intake in their class.

EXTENSION IDEA: Involve the entire school in this activity, assessing food intake in other classes and grade levels. You may even want to challenge another class to a "good nutrition" duel, setting goals, graphing progress, and rewarding completed goals with small prizes or incentives.

Create A Recipe

Devising a recipe gives kids a chance to develop measuring and writing skills, exercise their creativity, and eat the results of their labor! They can also share their own recipe with family and friends or start their own personal "cookbook." Below are some simple ideas for recipe development that kids are sure to succeed at.

Before you start, review the guidelines for safe classroom cooking advised in Appendix A.

For each recipe, provide a clean table with measuring cups and spoons, scale (optional), plastic knives and spoons, paper and pencils, plastic gloves, bowls filled with ingredients, and individual plates or bowls for students to create their recipe.

YOU WILL NEED:
- Clean work space
- Measuring cups and spoons
- Scale (optional)
- Plastic knives and spoons
- Paper and pencils
- Plastic gloves
- Bowls filled with ingredients (see text)
- Individual plates or bowls

Have students work in pairs, one as the cook and one as the recorder. After each recipe is complete, the children will switch roles.

When creating a recipe, it is important to start small, measuring a small amount at a time and then adding more as needed. Remind students that they can always add more but they are not allowed to subtract (It is not sanitary to dump ingredients back into the serving bowl.) Demonstrate how to accurately measure ingredients, using the plastic knife to level off the measuring cup or spoon. After students determine the "right" amount of an ingredient, the recorder's job is to write it down. Later at their desk, students can add instructions and complete the recipe.

TRAIL MIX: Provide ingredients such as raisins, dried berries, other dried fruit (chopped, if needed), peanuts, almonds, pumpkin seeds, sunflower seeds, wheat germ, and quick-cooking oatmeal.

YOGURT PARFAIT: Use clear plastic cups to make the parfaits. Instruct children to layer their parfait as they wish, using such ingredients as nonfat lemon or vanilla yogurt, grapenuts or wheat germ, berries, banana slices, and melon balls.

VEGETABLE SALAD: Big on nutrition and easy to assemble, creating a vegetable salad recipe is one way to entice kids to eat vegetables. Include familiar and predictable ingredients (lettuce, tomatoes, cucumbers, carrots) along with more novel choices such as sliced daikon radishes, jicama, sprouts, fresh spinach, colorful pepper slices, fresh sliced mushrooms, pea pods, green cauliflower, and sliced summer squash.

PERFECTLY PERSONAL PIZZA: Students learn to create their own pizza recipe, perfect for a quick mini-meal or snack. Using English muffin or bagel halves as the base, spread with tomato sauce, sprinkle on spices, add toppings and sprinkle with grated part-skim mozzarella cheese. Examples of toppings include chopped onions, pepper rings, sliced black or green olives, mushroom pieces, broccoli or cauliflower florets, tomato slices, chopped turkey or ham, and lean hamburger or ground turkey that has been browned and drained. Try spices such as oregano, garlic, basil, thyme, parsley, or marjoram.

To cook pizzas, bake at 400 degrees for 8-10 minutes or broil for 3-5 minutes.

Calculating Daily Nutrient Intake (Advanced Activity)

For students interested in calculating their precise intake of calories, fat, calcium, or other nutrients, there are a variety of resources available. The more laborious way to calculate nutrient intake is to use a resource such as _Bowes & Church's Food Values of Portions Commonly Used_, which includes nutrient information on over 8500 foods (See Appendix B).

For students who enjoy using computers, several programs are available that analyze dietary intake. Most programs also compare intake to a standard recommendation based on age, sex, and activity level. Data is usually presented in a variety of ways, including graphically. Although most programs are geared for students at the secondary level, many fourth and fifth graders possess the skills needed to use these programs. (See Appendix B, audiovisual resources, for catalogs that carry nutrient analysis software).

CHAPTER 7

SCIENCE

"Thank you for coming. I didn't know that (for) every pound we gain your heart has to beat an extra mile."–Mark

When my first grade daughter approached me about project ideas for her school science fair, I naturally thought of all the possibilities that related to nutrition (next time, perhaps, she'll ask her Dad!) The idea that sparked her interest the most was to survey her class and analyze their eating habits. By the time we finished this humble undertaking, she had gained skills in a variety of subject areas. She developed a simple questionnaire that her classmates used to record their diet for one day, analyzed and compared their daily diet with the *Food Guide Pyramid*, and presented her data graphically, using her best art skills to design, color and display her work.

Because nutrition is a science, the prospects for science activities are limitless. This chapter presents learning ideas in three areas: food in the body, the study of plants as food, and how kids can use the scientific method to conduct nutrition research.

Food In The Body

Nutrition is the science of how the body uses food. Even young children can gain an appreciation of how food is broken down and used inside the body. The food we eat goes through five stages of processing: digestion, absorption, circulation, metabolism, and excretion. Simple explanations with engaging experiments and activities will bring these concepts to life.

TASTE AND SMELL Our experience with food starts with our nose and tongue. The sensation of taste is actually a combination of smelling the food and using

TONGUE MAP

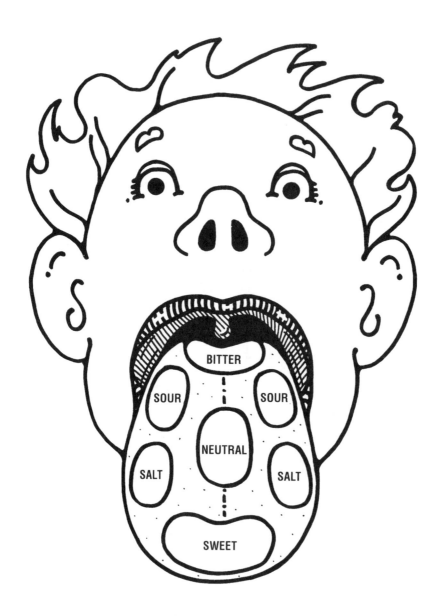

Enlarge and reproduce for educational use.

the tongue to detect flavors. Different areas of the tongue are responsible for picking up different sensations—salty, sweet, bitter, or sour, shown on the "tongue map" on page 76.

ACTIVITIES

• At snack or mealtime, instruct children to take a bite of one food and describe how it tastes. Next, have them hold their noses and take a bite of the same food. Ask them to describe the taste of the food and how it changed. Discuss how the sense of smell plays a part in detecting the flavor of foods.

• Students can learn to identify the different taste areas on the tongue. Supplies for this activity include cups of water, napkins, and small samples of food that represent each flavor: bittersweet chocolate, lemon, salted pretzels, and gum drops.

> **YOU WILL NEED:**
> ◆ Tongue map (page 76)
> ◆ Cups of water
> ◆ Napkins
> ◆ Small samples of:
> – bittersweet chocolate
> – lemon
> – salted pretzels
> – gum drops

Enlarge and reproduce the tongue map on page 76. Redraw the map on the board or make into an overhead transparency. Ask children to experiment by placing samples on various parts of their tongue and noting the flavor. Between each sample, students should take a sip of water and blot their tongues with a napkin. Ask children whether they can taste bitter foods on the salty area or sweet flavors on the sour area, etc.

DIGESTION is the process of breaking food down into millions of tiny pieces. Beginning in the mouth and ending in the toilet, food covers a route about 25 feet long, all inside the body! After the **mouth**, food travels to the **stomach** by way of a tube known as the **esophagus**. Most of the "action" of digestion occurs in the **small intestine**, a 20 foot long organ that completes digestion and transfers nutrients through its walls to the blood stream. In the **large intestine** (larger around, but much shorter in length than the small intestine), water is added to waste products, making a paste that can be excreted.

DIGESTIVE DIAGRAM

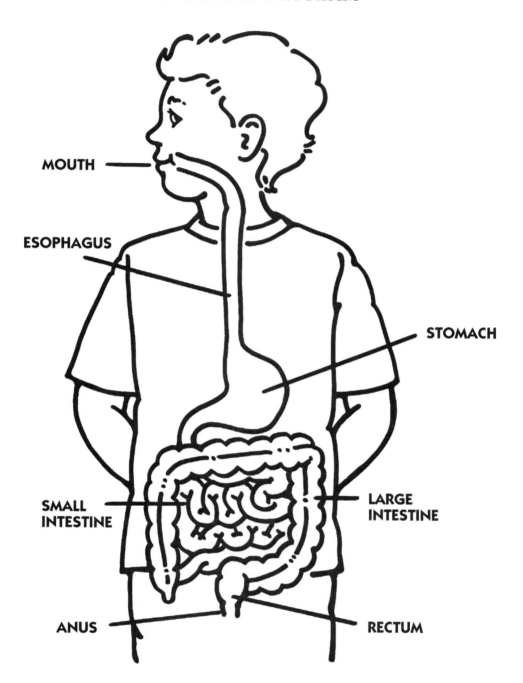

MOUTH

ESOPHAGUS

STOMACH

SMALL INTESTINE

LARGE INTESTINE

ANUS

RECTUM

Enlarge and reproduce for educational use.

While food is broken down somewhat by chewing and grinding, most digestion takes place by body chemicals. Chemicals known as **enzymes** break down food in the mouth, stomach, and small intestine. Other chemicals include **acid** in the stomach and bile (which helps break down fat) released into the intestine by the gall bladder.

ACTIVITIES

• Trace children's bodies onto large sheets of paper, similar to the activity on page 52. This time though, students will be concentrating on how they look on the inside. Enlarge, reproduce, or make page 78 into an overhead transparency. Ask students to draw and label the parts of the digestive tract on their life-sized silhouettes.

YOU WILL NEED:
- *Overhead transparency of page 78*
- *Large paper*
- *Tape measure*
- *String (25 feet per child)*

A digestive tract over 20 feet long in a child four feet tall? How could that be? Using a tape measure and string, have students measure 25 feet of string. Using their life-sized body silhouette, ask them to "fit" the digestive tract into the one they just drew, affixing it with glue if they wish.

• Even as we are enjoying the taste of food in our mouth, digestion is beginning. As the teeth grind and crush the food, an enzyme in the saliva begins breaking down carbohydrates into sugar. To demonstrate this concept, pass out small pieces of saltine crackers. Read the label, pointing out that saltines are made from flour and have little or no sugar. Ask students to hold the cracker on their tongues without chewing or swallowing. What do they taste? After

YOU WILL NEED:
- *Saltine crackers*
- *Napkins*

a few minutes, ask students whether the taste of the cracker has changed. Elicit possible explanations for this happening. Explain that the sweet taste means a chemical called an enzyme in their saliva has digested the starch to sugar.

Who was the first scientist to understand that body chemicals, not just mechanical action, are responsible for digestion? In 1822, an ambitious army doctor named Dr. William Beaumont was able to conduct digestion experiments on a living man! When fur trader Alexis St. Martin was shot in the stomach, he survived despite slim odds. But a small hole into his stomach never successfully healed, allowing Dr. Beaumont to conduct a multitude of digestive experiments and withdraw stomach acid for study. This fascinating story is told in *Dr. Beaumont and the man with the hole in his stomach*, by Sam and Beryl Epstein, Coward, McCann & Geoghegan, 1978. Read this book to the class or encourage intermediate students (3rd through 5th grade) to read and report on.

• The most slowly digested nutrient is fat. That is why a greasy meal can leave a person feeling stuffed for hours! One reason is that fat travels through the digestive system in big droplets or globules. When fat encounters the dark liquid **bile** in the small intestine, it is broken down into small droplets. Bile acts as an **emulsifier**, a substance that can break fats into small globules that will mix with water.

Using water, liquid vegetable oil, and a raw egg yolk, students can observe how bile breaks down fat during digestion. An egg yolk contains the emulsifier lecithin. (Lecithin is often added to salad dressings and other processed foods because it breaks up the fat particles, resulting in a smooth product.) In a clear glass, mix 1 cup water and 2 tablespoons of oil. What happens? Try stirring the mixture vigorously. Does the fat break down? Next, add the egg yolk to the mixture and stir. What happens to the fat droplets? This reaction is similar to how bile breaks down fat in the small intestine. (Incidentally, egg yolks do not work as emulsifiers in the body since they are changed by both cooking and stomach acid before they reach the small intestine).

YOU WILL NEED:
- Clear glass
- Water
- Vegetable oil
- Egg
- Tablespoon
- Spoon

ABSORPTION After food is digested into small particles, it must somehow move from the digestive tract to the rest of the body. That movement into the bloodstream is called **absorption** and happens mainly in the small intestine.

The small intestine is made up of millions of finger-like projections called **villi**. The villi are covered with a hair-like brush that traps the nutrients.

The nutrients are then passed through the villi into tiny blood vessels called **capillaries** which eventually empty into the body's major blood vessels.

ACTIVITIES

• To explain the concept of absorption visually, use a sample of shag carpet to illustrate the surface of the small intestine. Each fiber sticking out of the carpet is like a villi, ready to absorb nutrients and pass them into the bloodstream.

> **YOU WILL NEED:**
> ◆ *Shag carpet sample*

Readers of all ages will enjoy the whimsical story and delightful illustrations that depict digestion and absorption in *The Magic School Bus Inside the Human Body*, by Joanna Cole (Scholastic, 1989). Other titles of interest for young readers include *When I Eat*, by Mandy Suhr (Carolrhoda Books, 1992) and *What Happens to a Hamburger*, by Paul Showers (Crowell, 1985).

CIRCULATION How do nutrients find their way up to our nose and down to our toes? Every cell of the body requires a continuous supply of energy from nutrients and oxygen from the air we breathe. Oxygen and nutrients are transported to cells by **arteries** while **veins** carry carbon dioxide and waste products out of the cells. This network of blood vessels, including the small, weblike, connecting vessels known as **capillaries** make up the **circulatory system**. Our circulatory system relies on a very important pump, the **heart**, to continually move blood through the body.

ACTIVITIES

The hard-working heart needs good care to work at its best. Eating a pyramid-balanced lowfat diet, exercising, and controlling stress are all important heart-healthy habits to develop at a young age. Chapter 11 includes information and activities about the role diet and exercise play in keeping the heart healthy. *The American Heart Association* has a wide array of curricula designed to teach children about the heart and how to keep it healthy (See Appendix B).

METABOLISM Once nutrients finally make their way to the billions of tiny cells that make up the body, they are used to supply the building blocks for energy, healing, maintenance, and growth. Each cell of the body is like a tiny factory, taking the raw materials of nutrition and producing energy or growth and replacement parts. At any given moment, the cells of an active child are busy supplying energy to run at recess, creating new cells to make bones and muscles bigger, sending sugar to the working brain, and producing skin cells to heal a scraped knee.

Fortunately, the body does all these things without conscious effort. The only thing a healthy child really needs to think about is eating a diet that supplies the necessary raw materials.

ACTIVITIES

• What is hunger? It is the body's message to the brain that more nutrients are needed for growth, maintenance, repair, and energy. By the time hunger sets in, the body's energy stores are running low and the ability to focus on tasks becomes difficult. To illustrate this point, ask children to respond to their hunger in other ways than eating: by reading, doing math problems, taking a walk, etc. (if possible, delay their lunch period by 30 minutes in order to carry out this experiment).

Ask the children how they felt doing other activities when they were hungry. Were they able to concentrate? How was their energy level? Their mood? Discuss the role that nutrition plays in learning. Point out that kids who skip meals, especially breakfast, often don't learn as well as kids who eat regular meals.

Ask students if they know what the word "breakfast" means (break the fast). Explain that a fast is a period of time without food. Elicit how many hours their body normally "fasts" from suppertime to breakfast.

On the board, write the sentence "Breakfast is the most important meal of the day." Ask students to write or tell whether this statement is true and why or why not. Encourage them to write about their own experience with breakfast, including where and what they usually eat.

EXCRETION The final stop for food is the excretion of waste products. Even the most nutritious food has parts that cannot be digested and used, such as fiber.

After food leaves the **small intestine**, it enters the **large intestine** where water is added to form a paste that can be easily excreted. Other nutrient waste products are filtered through the kidneys and excreted through the urine (breakdown products of protein metabolism and salt, among others).

Plants as Food

Studying and growing edible plants is a wonderful way to reinforce nutrition and introduce children to scientific concepts and processes. Observation, prediction, and data collection are skills gained by applying science to gardening. A "growing" classroom or home can be as simple as a few seeds planted in a milk carton or as elaborate as a greenhouse or large outdoor garden plot.

Young botanists should be encouraged to keep a journal when studying and growing edible plants.

PHOTOSYNTHESIS A miracle really, life as we know it starts in the leaves of a plant. Using energy from the sun, carbon dioxide, and water, **chlorophyll**-containing cells in green plants manufacture carbohydrate. Plants comprise the first link of the **food chain**, providing food energy for other living organisms, including people!

ACTIVITY

• To observe the effects of photosynthesis, start with a green potted plant. Instruct children to observe, draw and record how the plant looks. Place it in a dark closet. Continue to water regularly but do not expose to light. Every two days, bring the plant out briefly to allow children to observe and record the

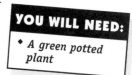

YOU WILL NEED:
◆ *A green potted plant*

changes. How does the plant change? Ask children to draw a conclusion about the effect light has on plants. Explain that photosynthesis cannot occur, thus the plant can make no food, when light is removed.

GERMINATION Even when dormant for a period of years, seeds will sprout when given the right conditions of warmth and moisture. This process is called **germination**.

ACTIVITIES

• To watch germination in action, place dry beans in a clear glass jar containing a moistened sponge. The sponge will keep the seeds moist and hold them against the side of the jar where they are visible. Ask children to carefully record or draw the germination process in their plant journals, including any predictions they make about the process or how long it will take. (And later, notes on whether their predictions came true and why or why not.)

YOU WILL NEED:
- Dry beans
- Clear glass jar
- Large sponge

Ask if anyone's seed sprouted "upside down" or "sideways." (the answer should be NO). Elicit from the students how seeds know to sprout "right side up." (ANSWER: Seeds respond to gravity by sprouting root down, stem and leaves up. This concept is known as **phototropism**).

• To grow edible sprouts, you will need small jars or clear plastic cups (baby food jars work great), clean 3-inch squares of nylon stocking, rubber bands, and 1 teaspoon of rinsed lentils or dry beans. Place the seeds in the jar and fill with water. Fasten the nylon square over the top with rubber band. Let soak overnight.

YOU WILL NEED:
- Small clear jars
- Clean, 3-inch squares of nylon stocking
- Rubber bands
- Lentils or dry beans

The next day, drain off water by turning the jar upside down until all the water shakes off. Rinse the seeds with cool water and drain again. Place the jar on its side in a dark place. Rinse the seeds twice a day and drain off water. Sprouts should be ready to eat in 3-5 days. For green sprouts, place them in a sunny window for one day. Eat and enjoy on salads, in sandwiches, or stir-fried with other vegetables.

GROWING VEGETABLES Potting soil or planting mix, empty milk cartons, and a sunny window (or grow light) will suffice for young gardeners just starting out. For classrooms who wish to garden on a grand scale, there are comprehensive programs available that assist schools in setting up a multi-grade, integrated gardening curriculum. The National Gardening Association has developed the indoor *GrowLab* program while the National Diffusion Network has published the highly-regarded *Life Lab* curriculum. Information on both of these programs and others is listed in Appendix B.

The activities below are designed to spark interest and encourage children to plant gardens at home. Most can be carried out with minimal time and expense.

ACTIVITIES

• Radishes are a great vegetable for the beginning gardener. Many varieties germinate in 4-7 days and are ready to eat in 25-28 days. First, fill cleaned half-pint milk cartons with potting soil. Read the seed packet instructions to find out the planting depth (usually 1/4 inch). Ask students to think of ways they can accurately measure the soil to arrive at the correct planting depth (a ruler or marked stick will work). Next, have students place 4-5 seeds in the soil (apart from each other), cover lightly, and gently water (To maximize drainage, poke a small hole in the bottom of the carton and place on a lid or in a tray).

YOU WILL NEED:
* Radish seeds
* Clean half-pint milk cartons
* Potting soil

Encourage students to describe the planting process in their journals. Ask children to predict when their seeds will germinate and how the seedlings will look when they first sprout. Every day, students can check on their plants and record any observations or changes. Keep plants moist but avoid over-watering.

Once the seedlings sprout, encourage students to make daily or weekly measurements and/or predictions about the growth and record in their plant journal. Results can be presented in a variety of ways—through drawings, tables, or graphs, for instance.

• The radishes should be thinned to two plants per carton. They are ready to pick and eat when the roots become round and begin to pop up out of the soil. After harvesting, weigh the radishes and record in plant journal. Wash, slice, and taste the radishes or use to make one of the radish garnishes described in Chapter 10.

• A great springtime gardening activity is to "start a salad." Students can then take their seedlings home and plant in a small garden patch or in large pots placed on their deck or patio.

Materials to start a salad include an empty paperboard egg carton, potting soil, and a variety of "salad" seeds. If possible, take the class on a fieldtrip to a garden center or nursery to choose seeds for this project. Examples include romaine, oakleaf, butternut, and redleaf lettuce varieties,

and spinach, watercress, and parsley. Fill egg carton compartments with potting soil and plant seeds according to package directions. When they have reached a height of 2 inches, send home with a note to parents, encouraging them to transplant outside or into a larger container. For easy transplanting, cut apart the compartments of the carton, poke a hole in the bottom of each compartment, and place in the soil, carton and all.

Encourage children to monitor the progress of their "salad" and record in their plant journals.

• Just like all living things, plants have a lifecycle. Growing lettuce can make a fascinating study of the lifecycle of a plant (which, incidentally, is my daughter's 1995 science project).

As a class project, plant and grow lettuce in a large container in the classroom. Observe and record progress of the plants and taste when the lettuce reaches maturity. Allow at least one of the plants to "go to seed," a process where the lettuce will produce long shoots with flowers. Eventually the flowers will form small seed pods. (This process, from start to finish,

takes a few months). Start all over again by harvesting and planting the seeds—a perpetual experiment!

Ask students why plants "go to seed," and why harvesting seems to prolong the process. Discuss the ways other fruits and vegetables produce seeds. Ask students to bring in examples from home (e.g. avocado pit, cantaloupe seeds) and experiment with planting.

PARTS OF PLANTS WE EAT The vegetables we commonly eat comprise a wide variety of "plant parts." There are six general classifications for edible plant parts including roots, stems, leaves, fruits, flowers and seeds. The activities below allow young botanists to classify, observe, and eat various parts of plants.

ACTIVITIES

• Explain that vegetables can be classified by the part of the plant they come from. The six general categories are roots, stems, leaves, fruits, flowers, and seeds. (NOTE: The classification of vegetable as the "fruit" part of the plant can be tricky. Explain that a "fruit" refers to the edible part that grows from a flower and contains seeds on the inside. The "fruits" that lack significant sweetness are generally classified as vegetables!) Brainstorm examples of vegetables in each category:

Roots: carrots, beets, radishes, (potatoes are technically tubers while onions are actually bulbs)

Stems: Celery, Asparagus

Leaves: Lettuce, spinach, cabbage

Fruits: Tomatoes, cucumbers, eggplants, squash, peppers

Flowers: Broccoli, cauliflower, artichoke

Seeds: Corns, peas, green beans

• Take a fieldtrip to a grocery market, farmer's market, or produce farm. Encourage children to take note of the variety of produce they see. Upon return to the classroom, make a list of the observed vegetables and name the part of the plant each comprises.

• Bring a variety of vegetables into the classroom for observation and tasting. Include less common varieties, including daikon radishes, broccoli-cauliflower hybrid, brussels sprouts, bok choy, and kale. Provide hand-held microscopes that students can use to examine the vegetables.

⊠ Make "plant-part art" for a snack. You will need large flat crackers, peanut butter or lowfat cream cheese,

YOU WILL NEED:

• Variety of vegetables
• Hand-held microscopes
• Cutting board and knife
• Plastic gloves
• Small plates or napkins

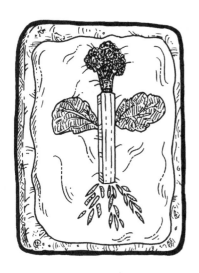

broccoli florets, celery sticks, lettuce leaves torn into small pieces, and shredded carrots. Students will first lightly spread crackers with either cream cheese or peanut butter. Next, they will create a plant or garden design using shredded carrots for roots, celery sticks for stems, lettuce for leaves, and broccoli

for flowers. This is an amazingly novel (and effective) way to get students to eat vegetables!

Using Science To Answer Food & Nutrition Questions

Children can practice using the scientific method and also learn answers to food and nutrition questions at school or home. The scientific method involves formulating a **question**, developing a **hypothesis**, coming up with a **method** or experiment to test the hypothesis, evaluating the **results**, and forming a **conclusion**. The hypothetical examples below illustrate how kids can apply this method to food and nutrition research. Students should also be encouraged to take the results of their experiments and use them to make recommendations for change.

Even very young scientists need to understand a few rules before setting up research experiments. It is important to get the permission of everyone involved, including cafeteria staff, administrators, students, and parents. Individuals should not be pressured or forced into participating and individual results should always be kept confidential.

GARBAGE AS SCIENTIFIC EVIDENCE Kids can monitor the cafeteria garbage to answer questions about what kids eat or throw away at lunchtime. The following example outlines one possibility for an experiment. Working in groups, students can come up with other ways of monitoring diets and influencing cafeteria choices by studying plate-waste.

Question Which fruit do second grade students eat more of: fresh grapes or canned pears?

Hypothesis Second grade students will eat more fresh grapes than they will canned pears.

Experiment Empty lunch trays will be checked on two different days, including one day when fresh grapes are on the menu and one day when canned pears are on the menu. Students will stand by the area where second graders return their dirty trays and record whether the fruit was eaten, partly eaten, or not eaten. The first twenty second graders who return their dirty trays will be studied each day.

Results On the day fresh grapes were served, 12 of the 20 second graders ate their entire serving, 5 ate part of their grapes, and 3 students did not eat any grapes. On the day canned pears were served, 6 of the 20 second graders ate their entire serving, 4 ate part of their serving, and 10 did not eat any pears.

Conclusion/Recommendation Hypothesis confirmed. Second graders prefer fresh grapes to canned pears. They ate more and wasted less on the day that fresh grapes were offered. The school lunch menu should offer fresh grapes more often and canned pears less often. Better yet, kids should get a choice of two or more fruits every day in order to eliminate waste and improve nutrition.

NOTE: Depending on the level of the students, the results can be manipulated mathematically, using graphs to plot raw results, or converted to percentages and presented in a table or graph.

FINDING OUT ABOUT OTHER PEOPLE'S DIETS Is it nosy to ask people what they eat? Maybe, but the government does it all the time when they conduct surveys of Americans' eating habits. Conducting nutrition surveys is a fun and informative way to learn about and compare the diets of different groups of people. Surveys can be descriptive, telling about the diet of a certain group of people, e.g. 8 year-old soccer players. Or a survey can be comparative, contrasting the difference in eating habits between two groups of people, e.g. soccer players vs. piano players. The example below is a comparative study.

Question Who eats or drinks more lowfat dairy products: third grade girls or third grade boys?

Hypothesis Third grade boys consume more lowfat dairy products than third grade girls do.

Experiment Design a simple checklist that includes the following foods: 1 cup lowfat milk (nonfat or 1%), 1 cup lowfat/nonfat yogurt, 1/2 cup frozen yogurt, 1/2 cup ice milk, 1 ounce lowfat cheese, and 1/2 cup cottage cheese. Ask third grade students to check off each serving of lowfat dairy products that they eat or drink for two days. Remind them to pay attention to the serving size, making one checkmark for each amount listed. (For example, if they eat 3 ounces of cheese at one sitting, that's three checkmarks!) Do not tell them you are comparing girls to boys—they may make a contest out of it, which will bias the results. Instead, explain that they should eat and drink just as they normally do. Collect the surveys after two days.

Results Fifteen girls and ten boys completed the survey. For the two days, the fifteen girls consumed 60 servings of lowfat dairy foods. The boys consumed 50 servings of lowfat dairy foods in two days. Using averages, the girls ate an average of 4 servings each in the two-day period (60 servings divided by 15 girls). The boys ate an average of 5 servings each in the two-day period (50 divided by 10 boys).

Conclusion Hypothesis confirmed. Third grade boys ate an average of 2.5 servings of lowfat dairy products each day while third grade girls ate an average of 2 servings of lowfat dairy products each day.

MORE IDEAS Once their mind is set in motion, students will enjoy using science to answer other food/nutrition questions. Encourage children to work cooperatively when planning and conducting their research. Perhaps the best gratification is that their projects can help initiate change in nutrition practices or policies.

Below is a brief list of other possibilities for nutrition research.

🎛 Working with the school cafeteria manager, set up taste tests with students for new nutritious foods offered by food manufacturers.

• Do a comparison study between kids who bring their lunch from home and those who eat at school.

• If candy sales are a common school fundraiser, offer to study whether selling nutritious snacks (pretzels, nuts, raisins, trail mix, animal crackers, etc.) can be just as profitable.

• Poll teachers in the school to see how many teach nutrition in their classrooms.

• Design a study to test whether breakfast cereals that put toys in the package contain more sugar than cereals without toys.

CHAPTER 8

SOCIAL STUDIES

"Your visit was FUN! Now I like vegetables more. My Mom and Grandma make Korean food—they make exotic animals! Since I was small my Grandma wanted to teach me it. Now they were impressed (by) what I learned!"–**Tara**

My childhood was filled with interesting food experiences, though I seldom appreciated their richness at the time. My Grandmother of German descent prepared the most marvelous pastries, homemade noodles, and Kraut Bieroch, a hamburger-cabbage mixture wrapped in delicious bread dough. My Father, the son of a Greek immigrant, practiced his heritage by cooking wonderful Greek dishes. The week before Dad made *Kapama'*, a chicken-based tomato dish served with ziti pasta and cheese, the whole house smelled (some might say stink) from drying goat cheese, usually feta or kefalotyri.

A major goal of this chapter is for children to appreciate how dietary habits and traditions vary between individuals and cultures. Children will learn to identify and evaluate their own dietary customs and explore the food habits of people in other cultures.

A unit on corn stresses the role that this grain played in history and the continuing importance of corn in modern-day America.

Guidance is given for students interested in studying the problem of hunger in their community. Exploring the issues surrounding hunger allows students to learn, offer solutions, and act to help those who lack access to nutritious food.

Identifying Individual Food Culture

Everyone eats, of course, but the what, where, when, and even how of eating vary tremendously. Children don't need to go far to appreciate the diversity in food traditions. Even within a single classroom, children can discover great variety in family food habits and customs. Besides differences in ethnic origin and religion, families make choices based on personal preference and convenience. The activities below will help students identify their own traditions and perhaps start a few new ones.

ACTIVITIES

Identifying Food Customs Ask students to think about the questions listed in worksheet 8-1 concerning their food environment. Encourage them to design and share projects that explain their answers in a creative way, e.g. by writing and illustrating a story about their family meals, designing a skit, developing a video of their family's mealtime traditions, or creating drawings, paintings, or posters which depict their family at mealtime.

Carrying the Message Home Be sure that children share their work and ideas with their family. Invite family members to visit, share recipes, and describe their own childhood food experiences. Consider hosting a potluck and recipe exchange which features food favorites from each family (check local health regulations and policies first).

Blending Food Traditions What happens when people from different cultures eat together? The book, _How My Parents Learned to Eat_, by Ina R. Friedman (Houghton Mifflin, 1984), explores how a Japanese woman and American sailor overcome insecurities about their different eating customs.

How different cultures use the same staple food—in this case, rice— is explored in the book _Everybody Cooks Rice_, by Norah Dooley (Carolrhoda Books, 1991).

Another book that explores differing perceptions about food traditions is _Family Dinner_, by Jane Cutler (Farrar, Straus, Giroux, 1991). Geared for the intermediate reader, this is the story of how a modern-day family who doesn't

Name _____

IDENTIFYING YOUR FOOD CUSTOMS

Everyone grows up with different food customs. The following questions will help you to identify your family's unique food culture.

1. Name and describe all the people in your family.

2. Does your family eat together? How often? Which meals?

3. Who decides what your family eats? Who shops? Who cooks? Who cleans up the mess?

4. Are there foods that your family especially likes to eat? Name and describe them.

5. What is your favorite food? Who makes this food? How often?

6. Are there special foods that your family eats on holidays or during religious celebrations?

7. Does your family sometimes eat foods that originated in another country?
   Name and describe.

8. Describe a meal or celebration with food that was especially fun or meaningful (e.g. Thanksgiving dinner, Bar Mitzvah, Birthday celebration).

9. Is there anything about your family's eating habits that you wish you could change? Describe the changes.

10. Fill in the blank: One tradition that I would like my family to begin is to
    _____. (Examples: eat breakfast together on Sundays, allow the kids to plan the menu once a week, turn the TV off at dinnertime, eat in a restaurant every other week, try foods from other countries once a month).

Enlarge and reproduce for educational use.

"do dinner" reacts to the efforts of visiting Great-Uncle Benson who insists "you can't have a family without a family dinner."

Food Cultures Around The World

Many different types and combinations of foods can be used to nourish the body. This becomes evident when studying various cultures and noting the differences in early native diets. But perhaps most interesting is the striking similarity in the nutritional composition of many native diets throughout the world.

Since the dawn of agriculture—roughly 10,000 years ago—people around the world have relied on a dietary staple rich in complex carbohydrate, most commonly a grain such as rice, corn, wheat, barley, sorghum, oats, buckwheat, or millet. In some cultures, the primary staple is a starchy root such as potatoes, yams, cassava (tapioca), and taro. According to anthropologist Sidney W. Mintz, these carbohydrate sources provide more than half of the world's calories, even today.

In addition to this dietary core of complex carbohydrate, most cultures include a high protein legume such as peas, beans, peanuts, chick-peas (garbanzo beans), or lentils. As Mintz explains, "This almost universal pattern in the diet of farmers is hard to explain; but whatever the reasons, it has been nutritively advantageous for our species."

Examples cited by Dr. Mintz include red beans and corn tortillas in Mexico, bean curd, mung beans, and rice in Japan, wheaten bread accompanied by hummous (chick-pea paste) in the Middle East, and in Caribbean countries, rice or millet paired with red or black beans.

ACTIVITIES

Learning About Dietary Staples Explain to children the concept of "dietary staple," i.e. the food that makes up the biggest piece of the diet, usually a carbohydrate such as grain or potatoes. Ask them why it is important to have a food rich in carbohydrate as the staple. (HINT: Take a look at the foundation of the *Food Guide Pyramid*). Ask if they recall the body's first and most important need, nutritionally speaking (Answer: Energy!—see page 35).

Discuss how cultures around the world have developed diets that are nutritionally similar, featuring grains or roots for carbohydrate and beans, lentils, or nuts for protein. Elicit reasons why different cultures living far apart managed to develop similar diets. (Point out that early agrarians needed carbohydrates as a staple because their lifestyle as physical laborers required a great deal of energy.)

Ask students to think and list examples of ethnic diets which feature a combination of grains and plant protein. Common examples include tortillas and beans from Mexico, beans and corn (a mixture known as succotash) from American Indians, and rice and bean curd (tofu) in Asian cultures.

Explain how diets around the world now rely on a larger variety of foods and many cultures, like that of the U.S., also rely on animal foods for protein, calcium, and other nutrients.

It's hard to characterize the "American diet," since the diversity of groups that comprise our culture has resulted in an interesting dietary blend. (For instance, where else besides the U.S. can you find "taco pizza?") Ask students how they think the rest of the world perceives the "American diet." (The probable answer is that American fast food, franchised throughout the world, is the perception of the U.S. diet by people in other countries).

What's Your Staple Carbohydrate? In this activity, students will keep a diet record for one to three days in order to identify if their diet has a staple grain or starchy root. Enlarge and reproduce worksheet 8-2 ("What's Your Staple?") on page 98 and pass out to students. Students will count the number of servings from each grain or starch and record on the worksheet. After they have completed the activity, ask them to draw conclusions and share with the class. While some may be able to identify one particular staple carbohydrate, many will notice that they eat a wide variety of grains and roots. Ask them how they think their diet differs from that of their early ancestors.

Name _____

WHAT'S YOUR STAPLE CARBOHYDRATE?

A staple refers to the food or foods that make up the biggest portion of a diet. Most early civilizations had a very limited diet that almost always centered on a staple which was high in carbohydrate.

Find out if you have a staple carbohydrate by keeping a record of what you eat for one to three days (using more than one day will give a more accurate picture of your diet). Record how many servings of carbohydrate-rich foods you eat in the proper spaces below.

NOTE: The standard serving size is listed beside each food. Be sure to take this size into account when counting your servings (e.g. If you eat 2 cups of pasta, that is equal to 4 servings).

WHEAT:
___ Pasta (1 serving = 1/2 cup) (e.g. macaroni, spaghetti, noodles)
___ Wheat Flakes Cereal (1 serving = 1 cup)
___ Bread (1 serving = 1 slice)
___ Bagel (1 serving = 1/2 bagel)
___ Hamburger Bun (1 serving = 1/2 bun)
___ English Muffin (1 serving = 1/2 muffin)
___ Flour Tortilla (1 serving = 1 10" tortilla)

OATS:
___ Oatmeal (1 serving = 1/2 cup cooked)   ___ Dry Oats Cereal (1 serving = 1 cup)

RICE:
___ Cooked Rice (1 serving = 1/2 cup)   ___ Crispy Rice Cereal (1 serving = 1 cup)

CORN:
___ Cooked Corn (1 serving = 1/2 cup)   ___ Corn Flakes (1 serving = 1 cup)
___ Corn Tortilla (1 serving = 1 10" tortilla)

POTATOES:
___ Baked Potato (1 serving = 1 medium)   ___ Mashed Potatoes (1 serving = 1/2 cup)
___ French Fries (1 serving = 12 medium)

OTHERS:
___ Barley (1 serving = 1/2 cup)   ___ Millet (1 serving = 1/2 cup)
___ Orzo (1 serving = 1/2 cup)   ___ Yams (1 serving = 1 medium or 1/2 cup)

___ _____   ___ _____

___ _____   ___ _____

After you complete this worksheet, answer the following questions:

1. Do you have one staple carbohydrate or do you rely on lots of different foods to supply your body with carbohydrates?

2. Why do you think people in early civilizations ate high carbohydrate diets?

3. Why is it important for you to eat a diet high in the types of carbohydrates listed on this worksheet?

Enlarge and reproduce for educational use.

Identifying Grains Collect grain samples, including common varieties (rice, oats, corn, wheat), a few that are lesser known (barley, millet, quinoa, triticale, etc), and as many of the corresponding flour or meal products as possible. Set up a center where students can identify and label the grain and flour samples. Provide a mortar and pestle so students can experiment with grinding the grain kernels.

YOU WILL NEED:

◆ Grain samples (see text for ideas)

◆ Variety of flour and meal products

◆ Mortar and pestle

World Food Map Display a large classroom-sized map of the world, labeling it "World Food Map." Assign students to research one country to determine a common food or group of foods eaten in this country. (This can simply be an extension of an assigned report on a particular country). They can find out this information by talking to people from this country, researching books, ethnic cookbooks, almanacs, and encyclopedias in the library, calling or visiting restaurants that feature food from their assigned country, or even writing to the country's embassy or consulate. An excellent resource, complete with interesting and authentic recipes, is *The Multicultural Cookbook for Students* by Carole Lisa Albyn and Lois Sinaiko Webb (Oryx Press, 1993). The following examples from the *Children's Britannica* illustrate one source of information that students can easily access:

- JAPAN: "Japanese-style meals include very little meat, butter, and cheese. The chief food is rice served in a bowl and eaten with chopsticks. A great deal of fish is eaten, sometimes raw, and other foods include pickled vegetables, bamboo shoots, bean-curd soup, sweet potatoes, and fruit".

- RUSSIA: "The chief item of Russian meals continues to be bread, which is usually of the 'black' (actually very dark brown) kind. Other traditional dishes are *shchi*, which is a cabbage soup, and *kasha*, a grain porridge. Specialties of Russian cooking are *pirozhk*i (little meat pies), *blini* (pancakes), *borsch* (beetroot soup), and various forms of sour milk and cream."

- ITALY: "The main meal, usually at midday, often begins with soup, which may contain rice, pasta, or greens. This is followed by meat or fish, cheese, and fruit. In parts of the Po valley, *polenta*, or cooked corn, is common and a lot of barley and chestnuts are eaten."

Give each child a 3" x 5" notecard to describe their assigned country's diet. They can do this in a variety of ways. They can write down the foods commonly eaten, draw a picture of the typical foods or an example of a meal, glue small pieces of dried food (rice, corn, beans, etc.) to the card, or create their own representation of the country's diet.

Allow each child to give a short report on what they learned about their assigned country's diet. With the help of the students, find the countries on the World Food Map and tack the notecards on the designated countries.

LESSON EXTENSION: Ask students to find and share a recipe for a food commonly eaten in their assigned countries.

• Plan a class party or celebration which includes an ethnic theme and food. Examples include African dishes at a Kwanzaa celebration, Mexican food for Cinco de Mayo, or a potlatch to celebrate Native American culture.

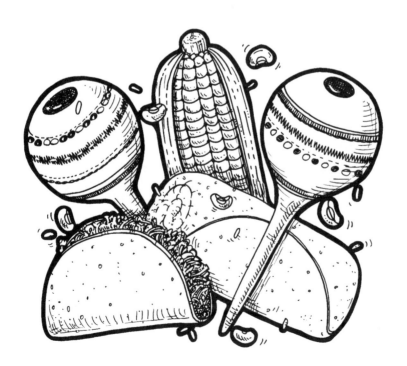

(IIl) Diversity in the School Cafeteria:

* Invite the school nutrition manager into the classroom to discuss how he/she plans menus which meet the needs and preferences of different ethnic groups in the school. For instance, some ethnic groups have a high incidence of lactose intolerance, which limits their ability to digest milk products. Other groups cannot eat pork or beef because of religious restrictions. Ask if there are ways that the school nutrition program accommodates these and other groups.

* Work with the school nutrition manager to plan menus and events which emphasize the ethnic diversity of the school community. Each month, a different grade or classroom could be assigned to develop a promotion for one ethnic group, complete with decorations, music, clothing or costumes, skits or dances, and of course, food.

* Offer to share recipes, food customs, and traditions of various cultures with the nutrition manager. Suggest ways that the cafeteria can integrate these foods into the monthly menu, perhaps by offering a rotating "ethnic bar" on a regular basis.

A Corn Unit

A grain with historical significance, the study of corn makes an ideal integrated unit. Besides discussing the nutritional contribution of corn, the history, modern-day uses, and experience by different cultures make a fascinating study.

READINGS Children will enjoy learning about the history and many uses of corn in _CORN: What it is, What it Does_, by Cynthia Kellogg (Greenwillow, 1989) and _Corn is Maize: The Gift of the Indians_, by Aliki (Crowell, 1976). High-quality color photographs show the modern-day production and harvesting in _Corn Belt Harvest_, by Raymond Bial (Houghton Mifflin, 1991).

HISTORY Corn, also called maize, is indigenous to the Americas, comprising the staple food of many early Native American tribes. Corn spread to the rest of the world only after Columbus landed in the West Indies and obtained corn from the

the natives he named the "Indians". The earliest American settlers would have starved if the natives had not given them corn to cook, eat, and grow. It was so valuable that the settlers used it instead of money to trade with the Indians for food and furs.

Most of the corn used by Native Americans was dried and ground into corn-meal using a flat stone called a metate, a job that was difficult and laborious. Today, powerful machinery in modern-day mills grind and process corn.

Eventually, the production and selling of corn became a way of life for many people who settled in what is now known as the "corn belt" of America (which includes Illinois, Indiana, Iowa, Kansas, Minnesota, Missouri, Nebraska, Ohio, and South Dakota).

ACTIVITIES

Obtain several ears of field (also known as dent) corn from a local mill or farmer. Set up centers where children can explore various aspects of corn:

YOU WILL NEED:
- Several ears of field (or dent) corn
- Mortar and pestle
- Clean half-pint milk cartons
- Potting soil
- Fish emulsion

• First, children can remove the husks and silk from the ears, a process known as husking. Ask students if they can name the state known as the "cornhusker state" (ANSWER: Nebraska). Next, they can shell the kernels from the cob for use in the following activities. Ask children if anyone knows the name of the machine that picks and shells large fields of corn (ANSWER: A combine).

Experiment with grinding the kernels. Provide a mortar and pestle, instructing students to grind one or two kernels at a time. (It's a difficult task!). Ask students to write or tell a story about how it must have felt to grind corn by hand, all day long for many days, like the native Americans once did (some remote tribes still do!)

Native Americans and early settlers used all parts of the corn, including the husks and cobs. Husks were used to make dolls and art, braided into masks, and stuffed into mattresses. Cobs were burned for fuel and made into corn-cob pipes. Ask students to brainstorm unique uses for cobs, husks, and silk. Encourage children to use them in creative art projects.

Using empty half-pint milk cartons, potting soil, and fish emulsion, plant 3-4 corn kernels in each carton. (Native Americans used fish to fertilize the soil when they planted corn). Observe and record the sprouting and growth of the corn plants (See chapter 7 for more on growing plants).

USES AND VARIETIES It would be difficult to make it through one day without experiencing a food or product made from corn. In the average supermarket, there are thousands of food items which contain corn. Besides the obvious— cornmeal, corn flakes, corn chips, popcorn, and grits—there are a multitude of products which contain corn syrup, corn oil, and cornstarch.

The biggest use for the corn grown in America is animal feed. Corn is also used to make many non-food items, ranging from tires and gasoline to glue, soap, medicines, cloth and many other products.

Although there are many varieties of corn, the three most common are field (also known as dent), sweet corn, and popcorn. Field corn is used for animal feed, ground into meal, and made into corn syrup, oil, and starch. Sweet corn is a softer, sweeter type of corn that is eaten fresh on the cob, frozen, and canned. Popcorn is eaten primarily as a snack food. Specialty corns gaining popularity include blue and white varieties, which are often made into gourmet corn chips.

ACTIVITIES

• Send students on a "corn hunt," either at home or at a local supermarket, checking ingredient labels to find products which contain some form of corn. Divide the products into two lists, one that includes foods that are primarily made from corn (e.g. cornnuts, corn tortillas, corn chex, hominy) and those which have corn-based additives such as corn syrup, dextrose, or corn starch (e.g. ketchup, pudding, soft drinks).

"CORNY" FOODS	
Main Ingredient	Corn Additives
Corn Flakes	Pudding
Corn Tortilla	Pancake Syrup
Hominy	Soda Pop
Popcorn	BBQ Sauce
Corn Oil	Gravy

🎯 Count how many items on the monthly school lunch menu contain some type of corn.

• Invite a corn farmer to speak to the class. Better yet, take a fieldtrip to his/her farm. Other possibilities include visiting a mill which grinds corn or a factory which processes corn.

• As a class, have a cooking/tasting party of corn recipes which represent various cultures. Examples include corn tortillas (Mexico), corn bread (Native American), and ugali (cornmeal porridge native to Kenya). Good sources for authentic recipes include _The Multicultural Cookbook for Students_ by Albyn and Webb (Oryx, 1993), _Native American Cooking: Foods of the Southwest Indian Nations_, by Lois Ellen Frank (Clarkson Potter, 1991), and _Spirit of the Harvest: North American Indian Cooking_, by Beverly Cox and Martin Jacobs (Stewart, Tabori, & Chang, 1991).

NUTRITION While corn is rich in complex carbohydrates and a good source of plant protein, it is far from a complete or perfect food. In the early 1900's, people in the U.S. who relied primarily on corn as their dietary staple often developed the disease Pellagra, caused by a deficiency of the B vitamin niacin. The disease had also been described in Italy and Spain as early as the 1700's. Interestingly enough, Indian and Mexican cultures who first soaked their corn in lye or lime avoided pellagra. (Scientists now understand that the lye reacts with corn to release the amino acid tryptophan, which the body can then transform into niacin.)

Using corn (or nearly any single food, for that matter) as an exclusive food inevitably leads to nutrient deficiencies. That is why the _Food Guide Pyramid_ is based on the premise that a variety of foods are needed for optimal nutrition.

Is corn a grain or a vegetable? That's difficult to answer, since Americans use it both ways, frequently serving frozen or canned sweet corn as a "vegetable." But from the standpoint of nutrition and botany, corn is best classified as a grain. (But why get picky?).

ACTIVITIES

• Students who enjoy library research can study and report on the disease pellagra, and how the U.S. Bureau of Public Health and doctors in the early 1900's finally solved the mystery of why people who ate mostly corn often developed this fatal disease. (A similar story to research and report is how a diet of polished rice led to the thiamine deficiency disease "beriberi.")

• ENRICHMENT IDEA: Students can note the nutritional contribution that various grains make to the diet through careful label reading. Suggest that students check the labels of whole wheat flour, corn flour, and oat flour to compare the levels of fiber, protein, iron and the B vitamins thiamin, riboflavin, and niacin in each product. Ask students to discuss which grain contributes the most nutrients to the diet.

> **YOU WILL NEED:**
> ♦ Label information from whole wheat flour, corn flour and oat flour

Helping Those In Need

Millions of Americans with limited resources go hungry each day. Faced with scarce pantries and empty refrigerators, many rely on community food banks and soup kitchens to make it through each month. Since food banks rely mostly on donations, the foods distributed through emergency food agencies are not always the most nutritious. According to one study, emergency food providers often fall short of dairy, fruit, vegetable, and lean-meat items.

All ages are touched by this problem, including an estimated 5.5 million U.S. children. Hunger in America often goes unnoticed because few develop the telltale signs of severe malnutrition—the wasted bodies and bloated bellies seen in drought and war-torn developing countries. While few American children are on the brink of starvation, many are unable to perform or learn well due to marginal nutrition and transient hunger. Virtually every community throughout America is touched by the problems of poverty and hunger.

Children can become involved by learning, participating, and offering solutions to the hunger problem in their community.

ACTIVITIES

• Invite a staff member from the local food bank, soup kitchen, or other community agency to speak about the problem of hunger. Ask the guest to describe the extent and impact of hunger, dispel myths about people who are hungry, describe efforts underway to solve the problem, and brainstorm with children ways they can contribute to the solution.

• Sponsor a school-wide "nutrition drive" for the hungry, emphasizing donations of healthful non-perishable foods. Brainstorm lists of canned and dry foods that fit the guidelines of the *Food Guide Pyramid*. Using the blank pyramid on page 40 as a model, create a drawing with examples of nutritious non-perishable donations. Send this list, along with information on the "nutrition drive," home with all students in the school. Be sure to include information on how people who lack enough nourishing food can find help in the community.

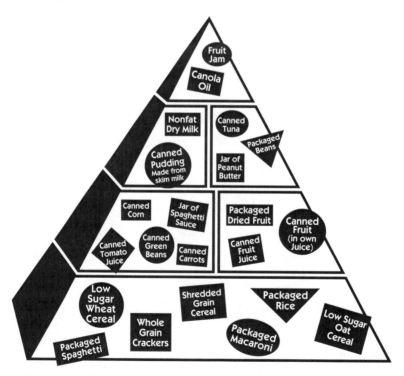

Suggestions for "Nutrition Drive" Donations

• To promote the "nutrition drive" to the school and community, plan activities that increase awareness of hunger issues. Students can create and perform a skit on hunger, make posters and flyers, decorate food barrels, or promote the drive through local supermarkets.

Enterprising young gardeners can raise money and awareness for hunger by selling vegetable and flower starts in the Spring. Start plants such as tomatoes, peppers, melons, or flowers in small pots indoors approximately eight weeks before the sale. (See chapter 7 for information on growing plants). Tie the sale in with another event, perhaps a Mother's Day tea, music program, field day, or other Spring school event. Working in groups, students can set up and decorate their plant stand, write an "advertisement" to send home to parents, and take turns staffing the stand. Students will gain practice in running a business and develop math skills by changing and counting money.

YOU WILL NEED:
- Small pots
- Potting soil
- Variety of flower and vegetable seeds

If the school has a community garden, consider donating fresh vegetables to agencies that serve those who are hungry or homeless. Children may also want to plant and grow vegetables over the summer in their home gardens. Encourage donations of extra garden produce to agencies who serve the hungry.

CHAPTER 9

PERFORMING ARTS

"Thank you for the radish spinners,
They were just a treat.
Thank you for the pickle fans,
They were sour but good to eat.
Thank you for the orange peeled rose,
That looks pretty while standing in a pose."

–Sweeta

Collaborating with a middle-school drama teacher proved to be a very gratifying experience. We worked with eighth grade drama students in the production of a nutrition play for elementary students. The idea was to motivate the younger children to try more healthful foods. I lent the nutrition expertise while teacher Adele White worked her magic, inspiring the students to create and perform a delightful 20-minute play. Using the costumed dog characters Sheggy Good-Grub (who eats well) and Sickly Spot (who subsists on "tip" foods), they enacted the consequences of nutrition choices in a play they titled "Sickly or Successful: You Decide."

The students performed the play for area elementary schools, leading the audience in exercises/stretching during intermission. The event was a huge success—the younger children were mesmerized during the play and nearly knocked Spot over (who transformed from "Sickly" to "Successful") after the play.

But the biggest surprise of all was the effect the process had on the actors. While eighth graders are not known for their great eating habits, these students actually began to take an interest in nutrition. (Granted, I did see cookies back stage a time or two). The big surprise came when I arranged a pizza party—with healthful vegetable pizza—and they gobbled it up!

Through the process of acting, role playing, and teaching others, students are able to internalize nutrition knowledge, making them more inclined to practice good eating habits.

Chapter four gives guidelines on setting up classroom dramatic play areas for children in the early grades. This chapter presents ideas on how to incorporate nutrition into performing art exercises and events. The children—so naturally dramatic and wonderfully creative, will inspire the best ideas—Please allow it!

Role Playing

Role playing in small familiar groups is a great way for children to "warm up" in a non-threatening environment. Use realistic scenarios that allow children to think critically and solve problems. Stress that there are no right or wrong answers but instead, the goal is to practice making choices and explore the consequences of those choices. Use the ideas listed in Table 9-1 or create your own.

Creating Food and Nutrition Ads

Creating their own food advertisements helps children to understand the motive behind the messages that blitz their everyday life. After reviewing the advertising techniques described below, set up activities that allow students to practice identifying these techniques in real ads. The final step is to use these methods to create positive ads touting healthy foods, nutrition and exercise, or other health-promoting habits.

TECHNIQUES USED IN ADVERTISING Advertisers use a variety of means to influence and persuade kids, many which are cleverly disguised as games or promotions. The list below describes some of the ways advertisers commonly market products to children.

Popular Characters or Celebrities Advertisers often appeal to the emotional attachment children have for a TV or movie character. Popular characters are licensed to sell a multitude of products—clothing, books, puzzles, toys, and yes, even cereal and snack foods. Likewise, popular celebrities are paid millions of dollars in endorsements to peddle soft drinks to kids.

TABLE 9-1

WHAT WOULD YOU DO?

Working in small groups, encourage children to develop and act out solutions to the following scenarios.

- Your friend thinks she is too fat so she decides to go on a diet that she found in one of her mom's magazines. She wants you to go on the diet, too. How would you handle this situation?

- After school, you always feel so hungry. When your mom's not looking, you grab a bunch of cookies and go outside to play. Later, you don't feel hungry for supper. What would you do next time you're hungry after school?

- You like it when your Dad packs fruit, vegetable sticks, and other healthy foods in your lunch. But the kids at school tease you about eating healthy foods, calling you "vegetable head." How would you solve this problem?

- Your friend says that a "Giggles" candy bar is healthy because the commercial on TV showed kids with lots of energy after they ate "Giggles". He is now convinced that "Giggles" will give him energy, too. What would you tell him?

- On school mornings, you would rather sleep longer and skip breakfast. You really aren't that hungry when you first wake up, anyway. But lately, you have noticed that after morning recess, you have a headache, your stomach growls, and it's hard to do your work. How would you solve this problem?

- You always have to rush to make it to afternoon soccer practice on time. You usually grab a can of pop and package of potato chips to eat on the way. The problem is, your stomach often starts hurting in the middle of practice, especially if you have to run a lot. What do you think is causing your stomach aches? What changes could you make to solve this problem?

- Your best friend is a picky eater who rarely eats from the five food groups. You have noticed that he looks pale and tired and gets sick a lot. What could you do to help your friend?

- Your mom is a health food nut. She is forever bringing home strange looking vegetables with even stranger-sounding names, things like bok choy, kohlrabi, and rutabaga! Worse yet, she expects you to eat them. You flatly refuse, saying you will not try anything that looks or sounds strange. Is there a better way to deal with this situation?

- Your big sister is pretty and popular but all she ever eats are salads and diet soft drinks. She says most other foods are "fattening." Is she right? What would you say to her?

- Your parents went out for the evening, leaving you with a teenage babysitter. She says you can have whatever you want for dinner, even candy! What foods would you choose?

Constant Exposure Marketing has become very sophisticated, barraging children with non-stop messages. Beyond television commercials, children may also be exposed to in-school promotions and company-sponsored curricula, kids'clubs with special promotions and glossy magazines, and product placements in movies and sporting events.

Exaggerated Health Benefits The nutrition or health benefit of foods marketed to children are often greatly exaggerated in advertisements. Products which contain little fruit are praised by dancing fruit characters or shown with images of real fruit. Candy bars are played up for their ability to "energize." Highly sweetened cereals claim to be "part of a nutritious breakfast."

"Free" Toys Many food products appeal to children because they feature free toys or sendaway products. These products are carefully placed in stores where kids will be sure to notice them.

Disguised Ads Advertisements in children's magazines are often cleverly disguised as comic strips, games, or puzzles. Kids often think they are just another feature in the magazine.

Wearable Advertisements Many children are unknowingly walking ads for products. Shirts, jackets, backpacks, water bottles, sports jerseys, and other everyday items often sport highly visible company logos.

ACTIVITIES

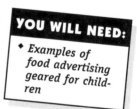

YOU WILL NEED:
- *Examples of food advertising geared for children*

• Ask children to bring in examples of advertising that use one of the techniques described above, including videotapes of commercials. Set up a center where students can identify and label the advertising technique, using Worksheet 9-1 on page 113 as a guide.

• For homework, ask students to watch at least one hour of children's programming on Saturday morning (excluding public television). Using worksheet 9-2 on page 115, have them keep track of how many food commercials they see. Based on what they know about nutrition, ask them to estimate whether the foods advertised are mostly healthful (i.e. one of the five food groups, reasonable in

Name _____

DISCOVERING THE MOTIVE BEHIND THE MESSAGE

This worksheet will help you to analyze how advertising and marketing influence the foods you buy (or ask your parents to buy). Use the checklist below to decide which methods are used to promote this product.

Food Advertised _____

Describe the advertisement (e.g. magazine ad, TV commercial, name or logo on a product, etc.) _____
_____

Check the categories below that apply to this food advertisement:

_____ **Popular Characters or Celebrities** (Does the ad feature popular sports figures, celebrities, or animated characters?) _____

_____ **Constant Exposure** (Is the product marketed in many different ways? Do you often see this product promoted on television, billboards, magazines, clothing, etc.?)
_____

_____ **Exaggerated Health Benefits** (Do the ads for this product try to make you think that the food is nutritious or a good source of energy?) _____

_____ **Disguised Ads** (Does this advertisement look like it could be part of the magazine? Is it presented in cartoon, puzzle, or story form so it doesn't look like an ad?)
_____

_____ **Wearable Advertisements** (Is the company name or logo on something you can wear or carry such as a shirt, jacket, backpack, or water bottle?) _____

Did this advertisement make you more likely to buy the product? _____

Do you think the claims made by this ad are true? Why or why not? _____
_____
_____

fat and sugar content) or primarily from the "fat, oils, and sweets" category. Ask them to note if there were any PSA's (public service announcements) that promoted healthful eating.

• Contrast the goals of the advertiser with those of the consumer. Explain that companies are in business to make money and advertising is an important way to let people know about their product. Advertising also supports television programs and magazines. Discuss or debate the merits of advertising, posing questions like "What responsibilities do advertisers have?" or "Should advertising be banned?" or "Should companies who advertise concern themselves with children's health?"

• For information on how to write to food companies or television networks, see "Writing Activities for the Young Nutrition Advocate" on page 60.

CREATING A COMMERCIAL Once children are familiar with the techniques used by advertisers, they can use this knowledge to create and perform their own 1-2 minute commercial for a nutritious diet, specific food, or other healthy habit like exercise. Working in small groups, children can follow the steps below to create and perform their ad—for the class, parents, or other students. In some school systems, students may even have the opportunity to record their commercial as a Public Service Announcement (PSA) for local television or radio stations. (The book, _Advertising: Media Story_, by Susan Wake, Garrett Educational Corporation, 1990, is a helpful tool for intermediate readers.)

Brainstorm As a group, decide which healthful food or idea about good eating that you want to "sell." Examples include a breakfast promotion, healthful snacking, a specific fruit or vegetable, "energy" foods, dairy foods for bone health, protein for a growing body, or the importance of label reading.

Create a Storyboard Working together, students will decide how to convince other kids to buy their product or take their advice. They will create a storyboard, which is the script for a commercial that contains both words and pictures. The storyboard tells all the specifics of the commercial, including details about music, actors, props, and timing.

Name _____

TAKING A LOOK AT SATURDAY MORNING FOOD ADS

To complete this activity, you will watch at least one hour of Saturday morning programming on a commercial network, such as ABC, CBS, NBC, Fox, or Nickelodeon. Once you decide on the channel, do not switch networks until you have finished this assignment.

NETWORK WATCHED _____

DATE WATCHED _____

WHAT TIME DID YOU START WATCHING? _____

WHAT TIME DID YOU STOP WATCHING? _____

Every time you see a food commercial, make a tally mark beside the category below that best describes the food advertised.

_____ Candy

_____ Pop

_____ Sweetened Beverages (not 100% fruit juice)

_____ Sweetened Cereal

_____ Corn Chips, Potato Chips, or other fried snacks

_____ Cakes, Cookies, or Pastries

_____ Sweetened fruit snacks

_____ Other sweetened foods

FOOD GROUPS:

_____ Grain (e.g. low-sugar cereals, waffles, pasta, rice)

_____ Fruit (fresh, frozen, or canned, 100% fruit juices)

_____ Vegetables (fresh, frozen, or canned, vegetable juices)

_____ Protein (e.g. meat, fish, chicken, beans, eggs, peanut butter)

_____ Dairy (e.g. milk, cheese, yogurt)

OTHERS:

_____ Combination Meals (e.g. children's frozen dinners)

_____ Fast food restaurants

_____ Public Service Announcements promoting good nutrition

_____ _____

_____ _____

How many total food advertisements did you see during the time you watched? _____

How many of these were for foods that you consider nutritious? _____

How many of these were for foods that are not the most nutritious? _____

Do you think there should be more advertisements for healthy foods on television? Why or why not? _____

Enlarge and reproduce for educational use.

Assign Roles Once the storyboard is done, the group will decide who is responsible for each role. Students must agree on who will act, direct, be in charge of music, design props, etc.

Design props or costumes Students can create simple costumes or props on their own or enlist the help of parent volunteers.

Rehearse Students should practice the commercial until they feel it is polished enough to perform in front of others. They may also need to make minor adjustments to the story board or adjust the length of the commercial (it should not exceed 2 minutes).

Perform the commercial Students can perform their ads for the class, other classes, the whole school during lunchtime, or as part of a parent program. Videotaping the commercial gives students the chance to critique and enjoy their work.

Evaluate the campaign Real advertisers want to know if their commercials work. Suggest students develop and pass out a simple questionnaire that asks the audience whether they are more inclined to try the food or suggestions just advertised.

Producing Skits and Plays

The possibilities are endless when it comes to developing skits and plays. Children can make and manipulate puppets, dress up as food, or act as great chefs hosting cooking shows. The ideas in this section are meant to spark kids' creativity.

RESOURCES Intermediate readers will enjoy the humorous account of the mishaps that occur during the class nutrition play in *Annie Pitts, Artichoke* by Diane deGroat (Simon & Schuster, 1992, see page 56 for description). Another excellent resource children will enjoy from the company *FOODPLAY* is the video *Janey Junkfood's Fresh Adventure*. An emmy-award winner, the program uses rap music, juggling, splashy graphics, and dynamic young actors to communicate important nutrition messages (See Appendix B).

SKITS A skit is a short play with a simple message. Skits range from impromptu classroom exercises (such as the role playing activity above) to productions which are elaborately planned and rehearsed.

At school, quick skits (15 minutes or less) can be used to promote an event or send an important message, as the examples below illustrate.

Work with the school cafeteria manager to promote a new food or menu. Perform a short skit in the cafeteria during each lunch period.

• Develop and perform a skit about hunger and its consequences to promote a food (or "nutrition") drive for the needy (see page 107).

Demonstrate the link between nutrition and exercise in a skit which promotes a school fun run, walk, field day, or other school-wide athletic event.

To promote environmental awareness, plan a skit which emphasizes nutritious foods with minimal packaging. Demonstrate how certain food scraps can be recycled to make compost (students will enjoy acting as worms, demonstrating the breakdown of food to soil).

PLAYS/VIDEO PRODUCTIONS A play or video production is often longer than a skit, and usually involves more preparation, backdrops, costumes, props and music. Some ideas:

A Pyramid Play Create a play about the *Food Guide Pyramid* such as "Chef Geometry Cooks a Pyramid," or "Food by Food: The Building of a Pyramid," or "It's Lonely at The Top: What it's Like to be a Gooey, Greasy Food."

The Evening News Build a play or video production around the theme of a news broadcast. Feature a late-breaking segment about how "label reading before eating alerts kids to possible nutrition dangers", human interest stories about kids who changed their life through a more healthful diet, cooking segments, an opinion-based commentary on food advertising, and on-the-scene coverage of the school cafeteria in operation.

Seasonal/Holiday Plays Put a nutrition twist on seasonal or holiday productions. Examples include "Goblins Who Gobble Good Goodies," "The Diet of the

Pilgrims," "Frosty the Snowman Melts Off Pounds," "How to be Sweet Without Sweets on Valentine's Day," "Why St. Patrick Likes His Greens," "Why Bunnies Don't Eat Chocolate," or "Nutrition and Your Teeth: Advice From the Tooth Fairy."

PUPPETRY Children enjoy manipulating puppets and inventing stories. A classroom puppet area or theater is a good place for students to express feelings and create dialog. To encourage scenes about nutrition and fitness, include food props, puppet-sized jump ropes, or personified food puppets. Kids enjoy making their own puppets, whether out of felt, paper bags, construction paper (finger puppets), or other material (See Appendix B for resources on puppet making).

Children will enjoy creating a traveling puppet play on health and nutrition that they can perform for younger children.

Teachers or nutrition professionals can also learn to use puppets effectively. It doesn't take a great deal of skill to tell a story with a puppet or two. The amazing thing is that children will automatically be drawn to the puppet on your hand, even though they realize the words come from you. Speaking through puppets gives adults a chance to express ideas and knowledge in a new, refreshing way. Kids respond differently to a message from a puppet, too. (That's why puppets are often used to promote open communication with children who have been abused or have emotional disorders).

Creativity Tips

Whether producing a commercial, play, video, skit, or puppet show, the following ideas are fun ways to communicate good-food messages.

• Interject humor by using food as edible props. Use a banana for a phone, carrot or cucumber for a conductor's baton, or fruit as juggling balls. An even more comical approach is for the character to eat the prop as they use them!

• A nice addition to a production is the use of poems about food or silly nutrition songs set to common tunes.

• Kids can play the part of life-sized food models. To help children "feel" the part, have a tasting party using real foods. As children taste apples, asparagus, french bread, or farmer's cheese, have them imagine how the texture, appearance, and flavor would transfer into a character role. An orange, for instance, may decide to act in a very sour manner, a cheese wedge might portray a mellow character, while grapes may decide to be very sweet.

• Puppets can be used as props within a play or video production. Food puppets can hover over a character's head, playing the role of the "conscience" which tries to convince kids why they should be eaten. A puppet show can also serve as an effective "play within a play," or as a television show or commercial set within a play.

CHAPTER 10

EDIBLE ART

"Thank you for showing us how to make those fruit 'sculptures.' Last night I asked my mom to buy some oranges and she did. I tried to make a rose but I didn't do it but I did better." –Krystal

More than mere cooks, many chefs are artists in their own right. Instead of paints and canvas or chisels and bronze, their medium is food and their tools are kitchen gadgets and knives. Like artists who make oceanside sand sculptures, the art created by chefs is transient, but beautiful nonetheless.

Chef Gordon McDonald knows how to work his magic on food, creating elaborate watermelon carvings, intricate garnishes, and beautifully displayed food platters. Along with Gordon and several of our young friends, we developed and tested many of the ideas that comprise this chapter.

The edible art ideas will capture the imagination of children as they delight in playing with their food. Some of the activities are easy while others require more practice. They are all designed with safety in mind—they can be completed using plastic serrated knives and other tools that are safe when handled properly.

Aside from the artistic merits of their work, children will also enjoy eating their creations!

As with any food activity, be sure to review the safety and sanitation guidelines outlined in Appendix A before beginning.

ZigZag Fruits

YOU WILL NEED: 1 piece of fruit per child (oranges, lemons, grapefruits, firm kiwifruit, or small melons), plastic ridged or semi-ridged knives, clean work surface and hands

DIRECTIONS: Cut a zigzag pattern (see diagram) completely around the circumference of the fruit, inserting knife to approximately the center of the fruit. For better control, instruct children to hold the knife approximately 1-1 1/2" from the tip as they cut.

Pull fruit apart to expose two fancy "crowns," suitable for a garnish or fancy snack.

Chef Tip: Different fruits can be stacked on top of each other to form a flower.

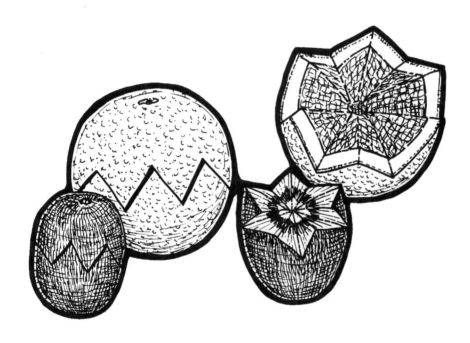

Creative Kebabs

YOU WILL NEED: long wooden skewers, colorful chunk of fruits or vegetables, clean work surface and hands

OPTIONAL: lowfat ranch dip (for vegetables) or lowfat vanilla yogurt (for fruits)

Suggested Fruits: slices/chunks of banana, kiwi, apple, pear, pineapple, melon, orange wedges, star fruit, papaya, strawberries (a spritz of orange or lemon juice will keep fruits such as bananas, apples, and kiwi from turning brown)

Suggested Vegetables: Slices/chunks of radishes, cucumber, cherry tomatoes, carrots, broccoli or cauliflower florets, mushrooms, pea pods, summer squash

DIRECTIONS: Create either fruit or vegetable kebabs by threading them onto a wooden skewer. Encourage creative use of color, design, and patterning. Discuss how kebabs could be arranged artfully on a platter, placing a bowl of suggested dip in the center.

Chef Tip: Make a bouquet-type display by inserting three or four kebabs into a raw potato half.

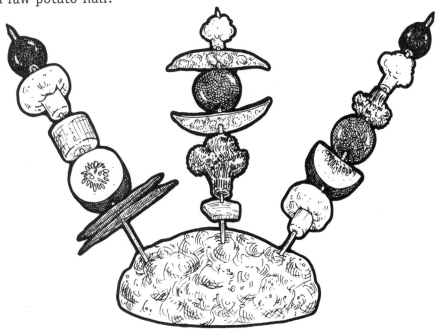

Food "Fans"

YOU WILL NEED: plastic ridged or semi-ridged knives, soft fruit or vegetable such as a fresh peach half, ripe fresh pear half, whole strawberry, or a large pickle or cucumber half for each child, clean work surface and hands

DIRECTIONS: Place food on work surface so that it is stable (cut "rounded" foods in half to prevent them from rolling). Starting approximately one-half inch from the top, make a length-wise cut completely through the fruit or pickle (see diagram). Make several cuts, parallel to the first one. Press down and "fan out."

Chef Tip: Cucumbers have a great success rate for this garnish. Try making the cuts at an angle across the cucumber for a different effect.

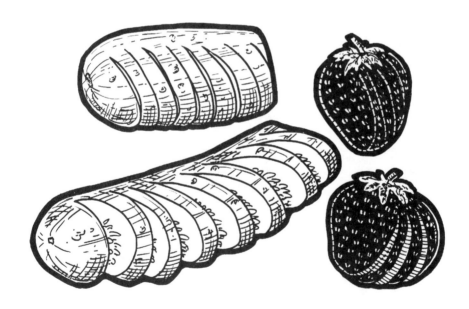

Baby Goose in a Nest

YOU WILL NEED: small or "baby" crooked neck squash, whole cloves, alfalfa sprouts, orange, plastic ridged or semi-ridged knives, clean work surface and hands

DIRECTIONS: Cut the orange in half, using the zigzag cut described on page 122. Carefully scoop and/or cut the edible contents out of the orange half, making sure to leave the peel in one piece. Create a "nest" by filling the orange peel with alfalfa sprouts.

Next, cut the squash off about an inch below the "neck." Insert whole cloves near the stem to make eyes (see diagram). Nestle the goose head and neck into the sprouts, so it appears the goose is poking out from his nest. If you wish, place two or three squash geese in each nest.

NOTE: Don't be wasteful! Be sure to eat the orange that was scooped out of the peel. The bottom portion of the squash can be sliced and eaten raw, cooked, or used in another project.

Chef Tip: Use small radishes or jelly beans for "eggs" in the nest.

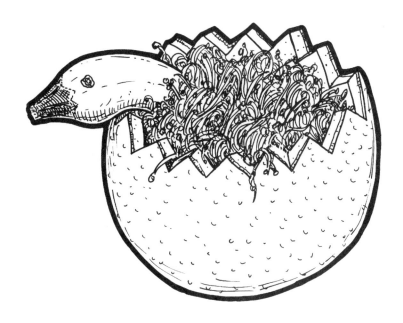

Radish Garnishes

Radishes are frequently used in garnishing because they are inexpensive, colorful, and versatile. They are also easy to grow—see chapter 7, page 85 for instructions. Three examples of radish garnishes are described below.

YOU WILL NEED: whole radishes, thinly sliced radishes, cherry tomatoes, lettuce leaves, whole cloves, uncooked spaghetti, plastic ridged or semi-ridged knives, clean work surface and hands

DIRECTIONS:

Radish Jacks: To make a jack, use two thin slices of radish. Make a single slit to the center point of each slice. Slip cut ends together to make a jack. To make a display of jacks and a ball, make several radish jacks and use a plump, round radish for the "ball."

Radish Caterpillar: Using thinly sliced radishes, arrange slices on a lettuce leaf, as shown in diagram. For a head, use a cherry tomato half with cloves for eyes and small pieces of broken spaghetti or carrot peeling for antennae. Use the same technique to make caterpillars out of sliced carrots or small cucumbers.

Chef Tip: White icicle radishes work great because they are long. Watch out though—these can be very hot!

Radish Mouse: Use a large whole radish with the root (which becomes the tail) still attached. Trim the stem, leaving a small stub for the nose. Use two thin radish slices from another radish for the ears. Make small slits on top of the "head," and insert ears. Use whole cloves for eyes and small pieces of broken spaghetti for whiskers.

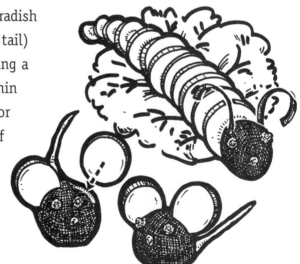

Sandwich Art

Use the following ideas to turn sandwiches into artwork that looks back at you!

HOAGIE FACES

YOU WILL NEED: hoagie buns, sliced lowfat cheese, lean luncheon or deli meat, shredded carrots, lettuce, or sprouts, olives, cherry tomatoes, miscellaneous condiments (mustard, reduced fat mayonnaise, etc), toothpicks (or broken spaghetti pieces), clean work surface and hands

DIRECTIONS: Make hoagie sandwich, using desired ingredients. On one end of the sandwich, use toothpicks or broken spaghetti pieces to position olives for eyeballs, and cherry tomato for nose. Arrange shredded carrots, lettuce, or sprouts on top for hair (see diagram). If desired, stick a small piece of lunch meat out of the "mouth" for a tongue. NOTE: Be sure to remove all toothpicks before eating!

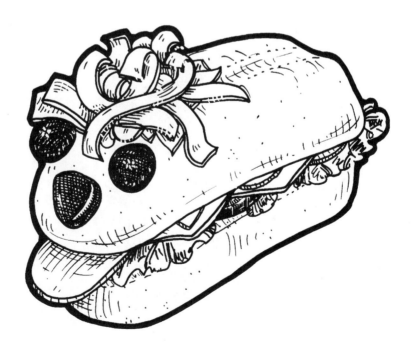

PIZZA FACES

YOU WILL NEED: English muffins (split open), prepared pizza or spaghetti sauce, grated part-skim mozzarella cheese, vegetables such as sliced olives, sliced mushrooms, red pepper rings, chopped onions, and broccoli florets, spoons, clean work surface and hands

DIRECTIONS: Spread English muffin half with pizza sauce and top with mozzarella cheese. Using the vegetables, create a "face" design. Broil 3-4 minutes or until cheese is golden and bubbly.

Chef Tip: Adapt this activity for special holidays. Make Jack-O'-Lantern, Santa, Cupid, or Leprechaun pizza faces!

FRESH FACES

YOU WILL NEED: English muffins (split open), peanut butter or reduced fat cream cheese, pineapple tidbits, sunflower seeds, raisins, alfalfa sprouts, plastic knives, clean work surface and hands

DIRECTIONS: Spread muffin half with peanut butter or cream cheese. Using remaining ingredients, make a face or other art design.

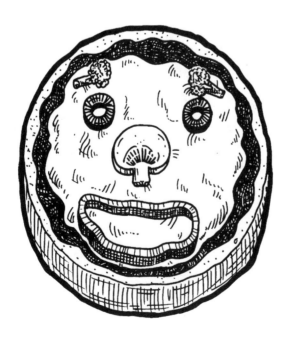

Bread Dough Art

Using bread dough, children can create virtually any shape, letter, animal, or design that they wish. It's as versatile as clay and a lot more delicious!

YOU WILL NEED: frozen bread dough (whole wheat is preferable), unbaked roll or bread dough from the school cafeteria, or bread dough from scratch; cookie sheet, parchment baking paper, clean work surface and hands

DIRECTIONS: If dough is frozen, thaw beforehand. On a floured surface, divide dough into individual portions. Pass out to children, instructing them to roll, knead, and shape dough into desired shape. Place on cookie sheet lined with parchment baking paper, labelling each childs' creation. Preheat oven to 375 degrees. Let rise, uncovered, for 15-20 minutes in a warm, draft-free place. Bake bread on center shelf of oven for 15-20 minutes (until golden brown). Cooking time will vary depending on shape and thickness of art.

OPTIONAL: Discuss the scientific principles involved in bread baking, including how yeast causes bread to rise and predictions about how the art will change during the baking process.

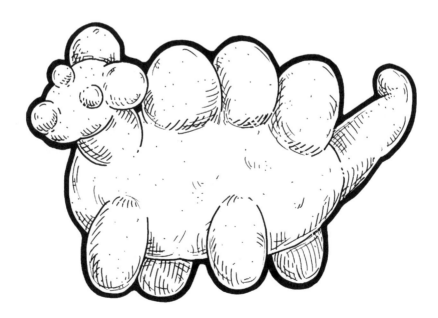

Pyramid Sculpture

Imagine a *Food Guide Pyramid* that you can actually eat! This 3-dimensional sculpture will remind children where each food group fits on the pyramid.

YOU WILL NEED: A thick slice of french bread, flat apple slice, flat cucumber slice, hard-boiled egg slices, cheese slices, reduced-fat cream cheese, chocolate candy "kiss," ridged or semi-ridged serrated knife, clean work surface and hands

DIRECTIONS: Assemble the pyramid with bread as the base, apple and cucumber slices on the next level, and cheese and egg slices on top. For the "tip," place the chocolate candy kiss on top.

OPTIONAL: Use reduced-fat cream cheese between the layers to hold the sculpture together.

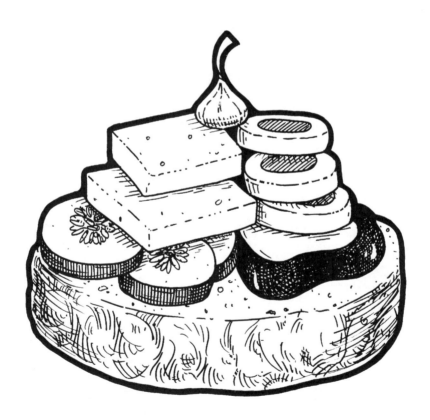

Cookie Cutter Fun

Cookie cutters can be used with food in many imaginative ways. Designs are especially fun when they complement thematic units or parties.

You don't even need actual cookie cutters—hunt the classroom or playroom for interesting plastic toys of varying shapes and sizes. As long as objects can be sanitized in hot, soapy water, they can be used for the following projects.

YOU WILL NEED: cookie cutters, plastic ridged or semi-ridged knives, foods of choice (see directions), clean work surface and hands

DIRECTIONS:

Fun Shaped Sandwiches: Cut sandwiches with soft fillings such as cheese, peanut butter, or tuna salad into fun shapes. Don't waste the outside edges—they can be cut into small finger sandwiches.

Breakfast Art: Use cookie cutters to make fun-shaped pancakes, waffles, or french toast.

Cheese Shapes: Cut cheese slices into various shapes and arrange on a platter with crackers. Or, melt cheese shapes onto dark bread or toast to make unique open-faced toasted cheese sandwiches (Children this age require supervision when using broiler or microwave oven).

Contrasting Cut-outs: Using either light and dark breads (light rye and pumpernickel work well) or white and orange cheeses, create contrasting designs with cookie cutters. Carefully cut identical sections out of both slices of cheese or bread. Insert the dark cut-out into the light piece and the light cut-out into the dark piece (see diagram).

Indentations: On the top of bread, sandwiches, pancakes, or sliced cake, press cookie cutter lightly until an indentation is visible.

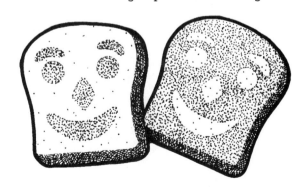

Expanding on Edible Art

The following ideas can be assigned as homework or included as suggestions in a parent newsletter.

• At home, encourage children to garnish a serving platter, salad bowl, or individual plates as a way to make family dinners extra special.

• Older children may want to host or "cater" an event for their friends. Birthday or holiday parties, post-game get togethers, or even "break the boredom" events are all chances for kids to impress their friends with their food savvy.

• Snacktime becomes learning and fun time when students prepare food in fancy ways. Children may actually eat a more varied diet when they have a hand in making it.

⊕ At school, students can make fancy garnishes for the cafeteria serving line or self-service variety bars.

• A visiting chef can teach students additional garnishes and cooking skills, expose children to careers in the culinary field, and reinforce nutrition concepts.

One program that outlines how to successfully teach nutrition through the culinary arts is *Nutrition From the Culinary View*, a curriculum for fourth and fifth graders which emphasizes that healthful foods must look and taste good, too! (See Appendix B for ordering information).

• Encourage children to expand their culinary skills by checking out one of the kids' cookbooks or garnishing books listed in Appendix B.

CHAPTER 11

PHYSICAL EDUCATION

"Thank you for coming to our class and baking bread with us. I made a dancer, because that's what I do in my spare time. Highland Dancing requires a lot of energy and endurance."–Joy

Food is only one part of the fitness equation. The optimal growth and development of young bodies requires movement, play, and exercise (rest, too!). A successful physical fitness program emphasizes fun, fitness, and life skills.

Children who are active feel better, have more energy, and even learn more easily than their sedentary peers. A strong physical education program, along with a solid nutrition program, boosts the entire school learning environment. Children in good physical condition bring more focus, stamina, and creativity to the classroom.

Nutrition principles are naturally integrated into the study and practice of physical education. This chapter includes activities which reinforce the role diet and exercise play in heart health, the importance of goal setting when targeting health behaviors, the best foods to eat for sports and play, active games which reinforce nutrition knowledge, and secrets from one teacher who integrates walking into all aspects of her curriculum.

Taking Care of the Hard-Working Heart

The strongest muscle in the body, the heart pumps over 2000 gallons of blood each day. Because it is a muscle, the heart becomes stronger and more efficient when it is exercised regularly.

Diet also plays a vital role in keeping the heart healthy. While nutrition scientists continue to search for definitive answers about diet and heart health, they do know that a high intake of cholesterol and saturated fat places many people at increased risk for heart disease (See Table 11-1 for "Fat Facts"). When the concentration of cholesterol in the blood runs consistently high, fatty deposits eventually build up in the **coronary arteries**, the blood vessels that supply the heart with oxygen and nutrients. When a coronary artery becomes completely blocked with fat, the blood supply in that section of the heart muscle is shut off, resulting in the life-threatening event known as a "heart attack."

THE HEART

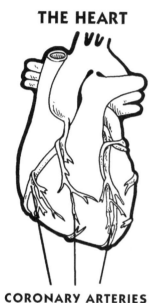

CORONARY ARTERIES

Limiting fat is only one piece of a heart smart lifestyle, though. Eating an overall well balanced diet—rich in high fiber grains, fruits and vegetables—lowers the risk of heart disease. Also vital to heart health are lifetime habits that include regular exercise, relaxation, a tobacco-free lifestyle, and the control of blood pressure.

While it is the rare child who will experience coronary heart disease in youth, autopsy studies demonstrate that the process leading to fatty arteries begins in childhood. Clearly, the best "cure" for heart disease involves adopting healthful habits early on.

PULSE RATE Teach children to monitor their pulse rate, using their index and middle fingers on either the wrist or neck (carotid pulse). An easy way to find the carotid pulse is to place the thumb of the right hand on the chin and then search with the first two fingers until the pulse feels strong and steady. Time the pulse for six seconds, instructing children when to start and stop counting. Multiply the number times 10 for the beats-per-minute pulse rate.

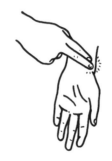
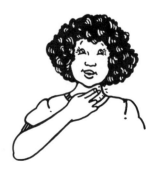

TABLE 11-1

FAT FACTS

- Fat is essential to health. In spite of all the bad press, fat is necessary, both on the body and in the diet:
  - In the body, fat serves as a shock absorber that protects internal organs, aids in temperature regulation, provides insulation, serves as an energy reservoir, and comprises an important part of the cell membrane.
  - In the diet, fat provides the essential fatty acid linoleic acid. Dietary fat also aids in the transport and absorption of the fat soluble vitamins (A, D, E, and K).
  - Fat plays an important role in promoting growth and development in infants. Breast milk, nature's perfect food for babies, derives over half of its calories from fat and is high in cholesterol as well.
  - Finally, fat tastes good and provides a feeling of satisfaction. Since fat is digested more slowly than carbohydrate or protein, it delays feelings of hunger between meals.
- Too much fat—both in the diet and on the body—creates problems for a large percentage of Americans. The rate and severity of obesity continues to rise for both children and adults (in spite of a multibillion dollar weight-loss industry). Americans eat approximately 34-37% of their calories from fat, although a more healthful 25-30% calories from fat is recommended.
- Fat is "fattening" in the sense that it contains nine calories per gram, while the other energy nutrients—carbohydrate and protein—each contain four calories per gram.
- Obesity is associated with many chronic health problems, including high blood pressure, mechanical stress on the joints, diabetes, heart disease, and certain types of cancer.
- Eating a diet high in fat increases the risk of colon, prostate, and (probably) breast cancer.
- A high level of cholesterol in the blood is a major risk factor for coronary artery disease. A blockage in an artery leading to the brain can cause a stroke while a blockage in the coronary arteries leads to heart attack.
- It is ironic and confusing that dietary cholesterol has only a moderate effect on blood cholesterol levels. The real culprit in raising blood cholesterol levels is the amount of saturated fat eaten. The types of fat are briefly described below.
  - Saturated fats are normally solid at room temperature and include the fats found in most animal products (meat, dairy products, and eggs) and certain vegetable oils (hydrogenated or partially hydrogenated oils, coconut oil, palm and palm kernel oil, and cocoa butter).
  - Monounsaturated fats such as olive oil, peanut oil, canola oil, many types of nuts, and avocados, tend to lower total blood cholesterol. Especially significant is their tendency to lower the damaging form of cholesterol contained in Low Density Lipoproteins (LDL) while preserving the so-called "good" cholesterol contained in High Density Lipoproteins (HDL). HDLs carry cholesterol from the coronary arteries back to the liver where it is broken down. (Exercise has also been shown to increase HDL levels.)

Table 11-1 continued on page 136

TABLE 11-1 — continued

FAT FACTS

- Polyunsaturated fats are also known to lower cholesterol and include such common oils as corn, safflower, soybean, and sunflower seed oils. Omega-3 fatty acids are a unique type of polyunsaturated fat that show promise in preventing heart disease. Fish, especially cold water varieties such as mackerel, salmon, and tuna, are rich in omega-3 fatty acids.

- Cholesterol is a waxy fat-like substance produced by the body and consumed in the diet. Blood cholesterol levels vary between individuals and are influenced by both genetics and diet. Dietary cholesterol is found only in animal foods. Full fat dairy products, egg yolks, animal fat, and liver are the most common sources of dietary cholesterol.

• Guidelines from the National Cholesterol Education Program recommend that children over the age of two average no more than 30% of their total calories from fat, 10% or less of their calories from saturated fat, and limit cholesterol to no more than 300 milligrams each day. The guidelines also advocate that children eat a wide variety of foods and consume enough calories to support growth and development.

• Not every single food eaten has to meet the guideline for 30% fat calories. It is the balance of the entire daily (or even weekly) diet that should register 30 percent or fewer fat calories. (See chapter 6 for information on calculating calories from fat.)

ACTIVITIES

• Contrast resting heart rate with active heart rate. (The resting heart rate for an average child is around 80 beats per minute.) Have children take their pulse at rest and record. Next, have them jump rope or run in place for 1-2 minutes, checking pulse immediately after they finish. What happens to the pulse rate?

• Ask students to keep a pulse rate chart, noting how their heart rate responds to different situations, i.e. waking up, after eating, when scared or nervous, before bed, during active play or exercise, etc.

Laqueesha's
Pulse Rate

When I wake up 73

At a scary movie 94

After riding my bike 120

Doing Homework 82

• Assign students math problems that use their pulse data. For instance, using resting pulse rate, calculate how many times the heart beats each day, week, month, etc. How many extra beats does 30 minutes of exercise or active play add to the total each day? Does the resting pulse rate vary between children in the class? Are there differences between girls and boys? Plot the results in a table or show graphically.

• Pose the following "challenge question" to students: Will a heart made strong through regular exercise beat faster or slower when at rest? (Answer: The resting heart rate is slower because a strong heart can pump more blood with fewer beats. Many endurance athletes have resting pulse rates as low as 40 beats per minute.)

• Target pulse rate is the heart rate to strive for during an aerobic workout such as running, jumping rope, swimming, biking, or in-line skating. To build a strong heart, it is recommended that children exercise at their target pulse rates (shown in Table 11-2) a minimum of 20 continuous minutes, three times weekly.

TABLE 11-2

TARGET PULSE RATE

Resting Rate	Target Rate
below 60	150
60-64	152
65-69	153
70-74	154
75-79	155
80-84	158
85-89	161
90 & above	163

Source: *Learning91, July/August 1991, by Bruce Fisher, Chris Hopper, and Kathy Munoz*

EATING FOR A HEALTHY HEART Discuss how the *Food Guide Pyramid* can be a helpful tool in planning a heart-healthy diet. Ask children to list choices from each food group that contribute to good heart health. Discuss how some choices in the dairy and protein group vary greatly in their cholesterol and saturated fat content (A common criticism of the *Food Guide Pyramid* is its failure to classify foods within groups according to fat content). For instance, contrast the fat content of skinless baked chicken vs. fried chicken, whole vs. 1% milk, ground beef vs. dried beans, or nonfat yogurt vs. cheese.

ACTIVITIES

• Using one of the blank pyramids on pages 40 or 41, have students design their version of a heart-healthy *Food Guide Pyramid*.

• Ask students why they think Nutrition Facts food labels contain information on saturated fat content. (ANSWER: saturated fat has the most direct link to high blood cholesterol level). Visit a grocery store or bring in a variety of food labels and compare saturated fat content. Examples include butter and

> **YOU WILL NEED:**
> ◆ Label information from a variety of foods

margarine (see chapter 6, page 68), different types of milk, a variety of cheeses, labels from meat products, and snack items such as cookies and crackers.

How Fat Clogs Arteries Utilize the classroom water table or rubber basins to emulate the process of how fat affects arteries. You will need clear plastic tubing, solid vegetable shortening, cotton swabs, and red food coloring. Fill the water table or basin with water; add red food coloring. Explain to the students that the water represents blood, the tubes are arteries, and the shortening is fat that deposits in the arteries. Children can play and experiment, noting how a dab of fat in the tubing impairs "blood flow," and what

> **YOU WILL NEED:**
> ◆ Clear, flexible tubing
> ◆ Solid vegetable shortening
> ◆ Cotton swabs
> ◆ Red food coloring
> ◆ Water table or rubber basin

happens when the tubing is totally blocked with fat. (Remind children that the process of fat accumulation in the arteries takes many years and is not the result of an occasional fatty meal).

Goal Setting

When making any kind of habit change, it's important to set a goal and keep track of progress. This is especially true for health behaviors, since they involve changing daily habits. Children, especially those younger than age 12, have a definite advantage since their lifetime habits are still under construction.

ACTIVITY

• Encourage children to set weekly health, nutrition, or fitness goals. It is important to record progress toward the goal, which can be as simple as a checkmark on a chart, a daily bar to color on a graph, or a simple entry in a health journal. Consider individual as well as classroom goals (see page 71 for examples).

Examples of individual goals might be to participate in active play after school at least 20 minutes, four days a week or choose a healthy after-school snack each day. Classroom goals might consist of 5 minutes of daily relaxation or a minimum of two 20-minute classroom walks each week.

Goals should be simple, achievable, and easy to measure. It is also important to reward achieved goals. Non-food rewards are best and can range from classroom privileges, stickers, bookmarks, and pencils to business-donated items such as movie passes, water bottles, or gift certificates.

Eating For Exercise

THE BEST FUEL Active kids do best when they fuel their bodies with a high-energy diet. During exercise, carbohydrate fuels the hard-working muscles via breakdown of **glycogen**, the storage form of carbohydrate which releases glucose during muscle work. The body also relies on a steady stream of blood glucose to fuel all body systems, even the brain.

The best way to replenish the body's carbohydrate stores is to eat a diet rich in grains, fruits and vegetables (especially starchy sources such as potatoes, corn, peas, and lima beans). The more active the child, the more carbohydrate is needed for re-fueling. Fatigue, "burn out," and lack of stamina can all be signs that body carbohydrate stores are low.

ACTIVITY

Create analogies between the active body and an automobile. Have the children expand and explain the similarities, using the following examples: Gasoline is to a car like (food) is to a body, a body that runs out of carbohydrate is like a car that runs out of (gasoline), filling a car with high-octane fuel is like feeding the athlete with a high (carbohydrate) diet, an engine is fueled by gasoline in the same way the working (muscles) are fueled by carbohydrates.

Encourage children to write and illustrate stories which show the analogy between fueling a car and feeding a body.

THE MOST IMPORTANT NUTRIENT Water is actually the nutrient of most immediate concern to the young athlete. During training or competition, thirst is not a good indicator of fluid needs. Not only will dehydration impair a child's performance, it also poses a severe, immediate health risk. Frequent water breaks, especially in warm weather, are a necessity. Each pound of water lost through sweat should be replaced with 16 ounces (2 cups) of fluid.

Kids should be encouraged to drink before, during, and after practice and events. Plain water is the best choice, since it is cheap and readily available. Sports drinks, with their relatively low sugar concentration, make suitable fluid replacements as well. Pop, juice, and other high-sugar beverages are not good choices because they slow the absorption of water from the stomach into the body.

ACTIVITIES

Weigh children prior to an active physical education class, a sporting event, or other physical activity, and again afterwards. Have each child calculate how much "weight" was lost. Explain that the weight change was due to water loss from perspiration. Ask children to calculate how much fluid they should drink to replace the loss. (For more accurate results, instruct children to use the restroom before weighing and monitor fluids consumed during the activity).

• Have students keep a record of fluid intake throughout the day. Include water, juice, milk, and soft drinks as well as less obvious sources such as flavored ices, soup, and other liquid foods. A minimum of 8 cups of fluid each day is recommended and the active child will need even more. Suggest students set goals related to their daily fluid intake.

During the busy school day, children often forget to drink fluids. Remind students to drink water at recess, before or after breaks, and at lunchtime.

PRE-EVENT EATING What and when a young athlete eats can influence the outcome of practice or the big game. The hard-working muscles should be well fueled for activity. This is accomplished with a meal that is eaten two to three hours prior to the start of an event. On practice days, a snack or light meal can be eaten up to one hour before.

It is best to have the stomach as empty as possible during physical activity. Normally, blood is diverted to the vessels surrounding the digestive tract right after eating. Likewise, physical activity requires a lion's share of the blood to supply exercising muscles with fuel and oxygen. Exercising with food in the stomach stages a competition between the muscles and digestive tract, resulting in poor physical performance as well as an upset stomach.

Foods high in complex carbohydrates, moderate in protein, and low in fat and sugar are ideal for pre-exercise meals. The energy in sugar is short-lived while greasy foods hang in the stomach for hours (See chapter 7, page 80 for explanation of fat digestion). Fluids should also be emphasized prior to physical activity.

Good nutrition is also important after the game. This is the time to replenish the body's stores of carbohydrate and other key nutrients with a healthful, balanced meal.

ACTIVITIES

• On the board or overhead, stage a "digestion race," where students determine which foods they think will take longer to leave their stomachs. Pair foods with identical serving sizes, but varying amounts of fat. Examples include pretzels vs. potato chips, a bagel vs. a donut, high fat vs. lowfat crackers, or ice cream vs. frozen yogurt.

Ask students to explain the differences between the two foods, noting which will take longer to digest and why. Share *Nutrition Facts* label information from the products with the students, asking them to note the fat content of the two foods. Discuss which food is better to eat prior to exercise.

• Assign students the task of planning a pre-competition meal. Meals must be high in carbohydrate, moderate in protein, low in fat, and paired with a beverage. Students can get ideas from the sample meals listed in Table 11-3.

TABLE 11-3

PRE-EXCERCISE MEALS

The simple-to-fix meals below are great before practice, games, or as light meals between events during an all-day competition. Pair them with a piece of fruit and lowfat milk or water.

• Pita Bread stuffed with tuna salad (made with light mayonnaise) tomato slice, and sprouts

• Bagel Sandwich made of lean turkey, lettuce leaf, and a dab of light mayonnaise

• English Muffin split and topped with pizza sauce, vegetables, and mozzarella cheese; Broil until melted.

• Pretzels or Pretzel Chips and string cheese

• Peanut Butter & Fruit Sandwich on whole wheat bread (try applesauce, sliced banana, or raisins)

• Baked Potato topped with reduced fat or fat-free salad dressing

• Tortilla stuffed with hot refried beans, a sprinkle of cheese, shredded lettuce, diced tomato, and salsa

Cat B Suggest that students interview a local athlete about his or her diet. The student should find out what the athlete typically eats in a day, favorite foods, meals eaten before competition, foods the athlete avoids, and any special food or nutrition habits that help the athlete to perform better. Ask the student to write a report and/or present the information to the class. (But keep in mind that sometimes even the best athletes don't always practice good nutrition!)

Food Games

Active games that promote nutrition concepts can be creative and fun. The following games reinforce the principles of the *Food Guide Pyramid* as students engage in active play. Encourage children to develop their own games that center on a food or nutrition theme.

ACTIVITIES

Let's Make a Meal Relay Reproduce the food group names on page 144, cut out, and place in a hat. Have each student draw a slip of paper from the hat. The objective is for students to form a relay team made up of five members, with each student on the team representing a different food group.

Explain that when you blow your whistle, students are to mingle, share with classmates which food group they represent, and organize into "complete meal" teams (Warning: This is a noisy game!) Once a team is assembled, each team member will run an assigned length, relay style. The first team to finish is the winner.

Build A Pyramid Scramble Similar to the meal relay, students will again draw food group slips out of a hat. The objective is for the students to scramble, organize, and line up in the formation of the *Food Guide Pyramid* as quickly as possible. (WARNING: It is not advised that students attempt a "stacked" pyramid). Use a stop watch to time the class, noting their improvement with subsequent efforts.

FOOD GROUPS

Reproduce, cut apart, and use in Food Group Games

GRAIN   VEGETABLE   FRUIT   DAIRY   PROTEIN   FATS, OILS, & SWEETS

GRAIN   VEGETABLE   FRUIT   DAIRY   PROTEIN   FATS, OILS, & SWEETS

GRAIN   VEGETABLE   FRUIT   DAIRY   PROTEIN   FATS, OILS, & SWEETS

GRAIN   VEGETABLE   FRUIT   DAIRY   PROTEIN   FATS, OILS, & SWEETS

GRAIN   VEGETABLE   FRUIT   DAIRY   PROTEIN   FATS, OILS, & SWEETS

GRAIN   VEGETABLE   FRUIT   DAIRY   PROTEIN   FATS, OILS, & SWEETS

GRAIN   VEGETABLE   FRUIT   DAIRY   PROTEIN   FATS, OILS, & SWEETS

GRAIN   VEGETABLE   FRUIT   DAIRY   PROTEIN   FATS, OILS, & SWEETS

GRAIN   VEGETABLE   FRUIT   DAIRY   PROTEIN   FATS, OILS, & SWEETS

GRAIN   VEGETABLE   FRUIT   DAIRY   PROTEIN   FATS, OILS, & SWEETS

GRAIN   VEGETABLE   FRUIT   DAIRY   PROTEIN   FATS, OILS, & SWEETS

GRAIN   VEGETABLE   FRUIT   DAIRY   PROTEIN   FATS, OILS, & SWEETS

Enlarge and reproduce for educational use.

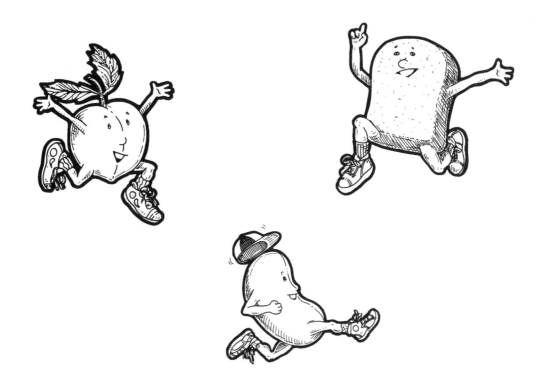

- **Jump Rope Jingles** Ask students to invent jingles with a nutrition twist. For example, "Food Guide Pyramid at my dinner, name each group and be the winner," followed by the child calling out a different food group for each jump (e.g. rice/jump, carrots/jump, peach/jump, chicken/jump, milk/jump). The goal is to name a food from a different food group with every jump (it's harder than it first appears!).

The Walking Classroom

According to Carolyn Johnson, a Portland, Oregon elementary teacher, "just about anything you teach in the classroom can be done on a walk."

Carolyn, a serious walker herself, "takes her classroom beyond four walls" by integrating walking into all areas of her curriculum. She divides walking into three categories: fitness walking, "taking a break" walking, and walking field trips and games.

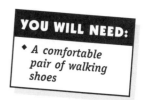

YOU WILL NEED:
- A comfortable pair of walking shoes

FITNESS WALKING When Carolyn takes her class on a fitness walk, she emphasizes a pace that is consistent, steady, and relatively uninterrupted. She works on warming up, cooling down, stretching, appropriate pacing, and good posture with her students. During fitness walks, she exposes her class to different walking paces and varying terrains.

On soggy Oregon days that are too wet for an outside walk, Carolyn sets up a classroom fitness circuit.

TAKE A BREAK Carolyn takes her class on short walks as a type of mental break. "Studies show that short walks can give us an energy boost and help to improve our mood," states Johnson. She gives her class walking breaks before an assembly when quiet sitting will be expected, when they need a "breather," and when they have been working hard and need a change of pace. She also walks with her class the first few minutes of each recess.

DISCOVERY WALKS Carolyn incorporates academics into walking by taking discovery field trips around the school neighborhood. Her students become meteorologists—observing, graphing, and measuring weather, evaporation rates of puddles, and creating big books based on their findings. They watch trees change throughout the seasons, note different colors, shapes, sounds, and different types of transportation. After a visit to a farm, her class walks to a neighborhood grocery store to see where the harvested food goes (and later develop a classroom grocery store based on their newfound knowledge).

Carolyn naturally incorporates her teaching of nutrition and healthy lifestyle habits into her classroom walks. "Perhaps the greatest reward from our daily walks is the growth of each child's self-esteem. Everyone is successful at walking and everyone has fun," she emphasizes.

CHAPTER 12

THE CAFETERIA AS NUTRITION LABORATORY

"I'm looking forward to coming and seeing the central kitchen. I like the food that your factory cooks."–Jonathan

As the nutrition lesson I was presenting came to a close, one of the first graders invited me to stay and eat lunch with her. Soon, several more children chimed in, pleading for me to be their guest in the school cafeteria. Curious to experience school lunch from a new perspective, I agreed.

As we crowded together to eat, I felt surrounded by adults giving directions over a microphone, pacing up and down the aisles, and hurrying each table off to play. My "classmates" warned me not to talk too much or too loudly. Before I had eaten half my meal, the cafeteria monitor excused our entire table! An eye-opening experience, lunch that day was a powerful reminder of how adult order and rules can sometimes bypass the needs of children.

Lunch is much more than a routine break in the middle of the school day. The cafeteria, at its best, *can* be an integral part of the education of students—offering children first-hand experience with nutritious food choices, a chance to socialize with friends, and a pleasant atmosphere to recharge body and mind.

This visionary cafeteria is possible but requires time, effort, and education to succeed. Training for nutrition staff, a commitment from school faculty and administration, and support from parents and the community all contribute to a successful school meal program.

Presented here are ideas on how every school cafeteria can become a center for nutrition education. Of primary importance is a menu which features choices consistent with the *Dietary Guidelines for Americans*. Students entering the cafeteria can then easily recognize the *Food Guide Pyramid* in action. This chapter also provides suggestions on how to enhance mealtime atmosphere and successfully market the school meal program.

For those worried about skin-tight budgets, the ideas outlined in this chapter make good business sense, too. A solid nutrition program—marketed right—increases participation and boosts image. School cafeterias throughout the country have successfully advanced their programs by making health-minded changes. A report released during the Fall of 1994 by the Public Voice for Food and Health Policy describes 41 school districts who successfully promote a healthful menu and nutrition education. (The report, *"Serving Up Success: Schools Making Nutrition a Priority"* can be obtained from Public Voice—see Appendix B).

School Meals: The National View

One goal of *Healthy People 2000*, the set of federal objectives for health promotion released in 1990, is to "increase to at least 90 percent the proportion of school lunch and breakfast services and child care food services with menus that are consistent with the nutrition principles in the *Dietary Guidelines for Americans*."

Yet, the 1993 *School Nutrition Dietary Assessment* (SNDA) study found that an average school lunch contains 38 percent calories from fat and 15 percent from saturated fat, nearly 1500 milligrams of sodium and a mere 47 percent of the calories from carbohydrate. Levels consistent with the *Dietary Guidelines for Americans* and *National Research Council's Diet and Health Recommendations* include 30 percent calories from fat, 10 percent calories from saturated fat, 800 milligrams of sodium (per lunch), and a carbohydrate intake of at least 55 percent of calories.

Clearly, changes must be made in the next five years if most schools are to meet the year 2000 goals. The USDA Child Nutrition Program, essentially the same since its inception in 1946, is long overdue for a nutritional makeover at the federal level.

A very significant development occurred in November of 1994 when the "Healthy Meals for Healthy Americans Act of 1994" was signed into law. This legislation will mandate the implementation of the Dietary Guidelines by 1996 (some states may have until 1998 for full implementation). The new law will allow those who administer school nutrition programs to choose between a revised food-based system or one of USDA's newly devised nutrient-based menu systems, "NuMenus" or "Assisted NuMenus." (To obtain the latest on these menu systems, contact the *Healthy School Meals Resource System* listed on page 177 in Appendix B).

But ultimately, it's up to each individual school to make significant progress toward the *Healthy People 2000* goals, promoting healthy school food services as well as the goals pertaining to school health education.

Nutrition in the Cafeteria

IMPLEMENTING THE DIETARY GUIDELINES Using the *Dietary Guidelines for Americans* to plan and prepare school meals is not difficult, especially if changes are made gradually. Involving students in the process is more likely to result in a successful transition (see "Ask the Students" section below).

Technical assistance is available to programs seeking healthful changes. Child Nutrition personnel at the state level can often serve as technical consultants and trainers for schools implementing a healthful menu and nutrition education program. Appendix B lists organizations that provide school food-service professionals with menus, recipes, and other resources useful in implementing the dietary guidelines.

School meal programs throughout the country are as diverse and varied as the individuals they serve. But in spite of cultural, geographical, and ethnic differences, all schools can succeed at making the cafeteria a healthful environment. Table 12-1 lists easy-to-implement changes that make a big nutritional difference in the menu.

OFFER CHOICE & VARIETY From clothing to entertainment to careers, today's children have a multitude of choices compared to previous generations. The same is true for food—children want a say in what they eat.

TABLE 12-1

15 STEPS TOWARD THE DIETARY GUIDELINES

1. Use nonfat yogurt as the base for fruit and vegetable dips, salad dressings, tartar sauce, and breakfast toppings. Besides lowering the fat in these products, yogurt adds calcium, protein, and other nutrients.

2. Substitute reduced fat mayonnaise for the full-fat variety. The reduced fat variety tastes nearly the same and contains about half the fat as regular mayo.

3. Increase the fiber in baked products by using whole wheat flour. If acceptance is a problem, begin by using a small amount in a recipe (25%), gradually increasing the ratio of whole wheat to white flour. Another way to boost fiber and nutrients is to add wheat germ, bran, or bulgur to baked goods.

4. Always have several fruit and vegetable choices available, particularly the fresh varieties. Purchase canned fruits packed in water or fruit juice. When cooking vegetables, lightly steam to preserve quality and nutrients.

5. Experiment with lower fat cheeses. Part-skim mozzarella is well accepted and can be used on pizza, in Mexican dishes, and sliced for sandwiches. Test different varieties of reduced fat cheddar and American to find brands that are acceptable in taste and texture.

6. Reduce the amount of butter used in cooking. Vegetables and rolls don't need to be slathered with gobs of butter. This is one "free" commodity that can have a big health cost if over-used.

7. When serving pizza, always offer at least one vegetarian choice. Experiment with new vegetable combinations such as pepper rings, broccoli florets, shredded carrots, or chopped spinach. Layer vegetables on top of sauce, then cover with cheese—a sneaky way to get kids to eat their vegetables!

8. Use the leanest ground meat available, whether lean beef or turkey. Always drain after browning (rinsing with hot water removes even more fat without loss of quality).

9. Plant flowers in the deep fryer! Prepare most foods by oven baking, broiling, or steaming.

10. Limit the choice of hot dogs and corn dogs—high in both fat and salt—to no more than once a month.

11. Merchandise low fat milk (1% or lower) as the milk of choice (although other milks can still be offered).

12. Remove salt shakers from lunchroom tables.

13. Offer nutritious breakfast items that are low in sugar, such as english muffins, bagels, low-sugar cold cereals, and toast. Reserve high sugar muffins, sweet rolls, and donuts as occasional choices. Purchase reduced sugar syrup for pancakes, french toast, and waffles. Other nutritious breakfast choices include yogurt, fresh fruit, and leftover pizza or sandwiches.

14. Write purchasing specifications with nutrition in mind. Clearly state the upper limits of fat, sodium, sugar, etc. that you define as acceptable in a particular product. Insist that nutritionally modified products meet taste and quality standards.

15. Work with manufacturers to develop and offer nutritious products that are acceptable to children. Offer to test and evaluate new items in your program.

Schools can devise a system of variety and choice that improves nutrition habits and reduces waste. A number of school districts have successfully implemented this type of system at the elementary level, offering a choice of three or more entrees and self-serve variety bars which feature a wide selection of fruits, vegetables, and breads.

One Oregon school (North Plains Elementary) witnessed particularly dramatic changes after the implementation of the choice system. Average daily lunch participation increased from 61 percent to 73 percent, the produce order jumped from 40 to 100 pounds per week, and the amount of food left uneaten on the average tray dropped 47 percent. By keeping an eye on the garbage cans and adjusting production accordingly, the school actually saw the average food cost per meal drop from $0.85 to $0.71. Because students were self-selecting much of their lunch, serving time was ultimately reduced (once children got the "hang" of it) and labor costs held steady.

A cafeteria that features variety and choice also provides options for children who are vegetarian, have specific ethnic preferences, or have medical conditions such as diabetes, food allergies, or lactose intolerance.

Guidelines for implementing this type of system are included in Table 12-2.

ASK THE STUDENTS! When making menu changes, the best "consultants" you can obtain are free and readily available—they are the students you serve each day. When kids feel ownership in the meal program, they are more likely to support and patronize school breakfast and lunch. Revamping the menu without the students' knowledge or support can potentially be a recipe for disaster.

Since food becomes nutrition only after it is eaten, menu changes should reflect students' food preferences. One way to elicit this information is to form student advisory groups. Some schools refer to these as Youth Advisory Councils (YAC's) or Nutrition Advisory Councils (NAC's). (For information on how your NAC can become nationally chartered, contact the American School Food Service Association, listed in Appendix B).

TABLE 12-2

TIPS FOR IMPLEMENTING A SELF-SERVE CHOICE SYSTEM*

- Plan the physical design of the new system. Evaluate and order equipment and supplies as needed (e.g. self-serve bars matched to student height, bread baskets, trays, tongs, etc.). Make sure the cafeteria layout includes space for an adult to monitor trays at the end of the service area.

- Offer a variety of nutritious choices of all food components. Consider offering standard choices along with rotating choices each day. Fresh fruits and vegetables are generally more popular than the cooked or canned varieties.

- Education is central to the success of this program! Nutrition staff, teachers, and administrators should be well prepared to explain the rationale and procedure of the new system to students. Parents should receive written information detailing the new program, including an invitation to eat lunch with their child (Consider hosting a "grand opening" to highlight the program 2-3 weeks after its inception).

- Be prepared for challenges and possibly extra labor in the first few days. Stock up on extra fruits, vegetables, breads, and other "variety bar" items.

- Integrate the cafeteria changes into classroom education. Highlight how this program positively impacts nutrition, meets the needs of more students, and how the reduction in food waste is good for the environment.

The guidelines in this table are adapted from a report prepared by Harding Lawson Associates (HLA), a private environmental engineering firm that conducted waste prevention pilot projects at three Oregon elementary schools.

Education is the key to making advisory councils work effectively. Students should first gain a clear understanding of the goals of the school meal program, i.e. to provide a variety of nutritious foods that students will eat and to operate the program in a cost effective manner. Ideally, students selected for the council will have some basic understanding of nutrition and why it is important. If not, this may be an ideal forum for hands-on nutrition education activities.

Children can also gain skills in constructive criticism and problem solving. Some students may be reluctant to offer feedback, while others may present a very negative picture of the school cafeteria (we've all heard the jokes and negative comments). A sample dialog that I have used successfully with students is included in table 12-3.

TABLE 12-3

TEACHING CONSTRUCTIVE CRITICISM

Students, particularly those in the intermediate grades, may resort to negative remarks when describing the food served at school. Responding to students in a defensive and critical manner only serves to worsen the situation. Below is a sample dialog that illustrates how to diffuse the situation and promote cooperative problem solving.

LEADER: Would anyone like to share their thoughts about the school breakfast or lunch program?

STUDENT 1: It's so-o-o-o-o gross!

STUDENT 2: Yea, I wouldn't feed that nasty junk to my dog!

LEADER: What I think I'm hearing is that some of you dislike the food served in the cafeteria. The problem is, I haven't heard much useful information so far. Right now, if I were to sit down and plan next month's menu, the comments I just heard sure wouldn't help me much.

STUDENT 3: I have a complaint—sometimes when I eat the third lunch period, the milk has been sitting out for awhile and it's warm.

LEADER: Thank you. It helps when you give me a specific example of a problem that you see in the cafeteria. You have a valid point—milk should not sit at room temperature for that length of time. Do any of you have suggestions on how to solve this problem?

STUDENT 4: Maybe you could keep cartons of milk in a bowl filled with ice.

STUDENT 5: How about using one of those refrigerators that can be rolled into the cafeteria at lunchtime?

LEADER: Those are great suggestions, students. In fact, I'm going to start a list of your ideas that I can use in my planning.

STUDENT 1: Do you think you could do something so that the broccoli isn't mushy? My mom always serves it raw with ranch dip. I like it that way.

STUDENT 2: And I wish we could have a salad bar more often. I always eat lunch the days we have a salad bar.

LEADER: Thank you, students. It is very helpful when you give specific examples and useful suggestions. With your help, I can make changes that improve the program for everyone...

Role of the Advisory Council The advisory council can participate in the school meal program in a variety of ways. Examples of NAC activities are outlined below.

• Poll the student body to find out the most and least favorite foods served at school. Brainstorm ways that favorite foods can be modified to meet the *Dietary Guidelines for Americans*.

• Conduct plate waste studies to determine which foods are consistently thrown out, uneaten (See chapter 7, page 88 for an example).

• Taste test and evaluate new recipes, commodity, or vendor food items that have been nutritionally "improved" (i.e. reduced in fat, salt, or sugar, whole wheat flour substituted for white, fortified with calcium, etc).

• Plan a menu once a month, designating it as "NAC" or "YAC" day. To give students real-world experience, teach them to cost out the menu and perform a nutritional analysis of their chosen meal, making adjustments as needed.

• Train advisory council members as peer educators. Provide them with simple lesson ideas that they can teach in classrooms around the school. Suggest they develop and perform a noontime skit on good nutrition for the student body (See chapter 9).

• Enlist the advisory council's help in devising a marketing scheme. Involve members in the development of a cafeteria slogan, logo, mascot, or catchy name for the cafeteria.

• Give the advisory council space on the menu for a "student's corner" where they can provide tips about nutrition and facts about the school meal program.

• Be sure to acknowledge and reward the work of the advisory council. Award students with special privileges, certificates, or small prizes such as pencils, pads, and stickers.

COMPETITIVE FOODS—TAKING A STAND The availability of competitive foods, i.e. foods with low nutrient density that are available for sale during the school day, undermines nutrition and health goals. When children can choose between a candy bar from the school store or a healthful lunch in the cafeteria, too often the candy bar will win out.

The issue of competitive foods is complex, often evoking debate among school foodservice providers, administrators, and even parent groups. In times of stretched budgets, school groups, athletic teams, and administrators resort to the sale of candy, pop, fried chips, and other low-nutrition foods—often through vending machines—to boost revenues.

While some states and school districts have official policies banning or restricting competitive foods, many schools choose to ignore the issue, fearful of "rocking the boat."

Unpopular as the issue may be, it is important to highlight the competitive food issue in each school. At the very least, a compromise should be agreed on and enforced that limits the sale of foods with low nutrient density to after school or during sporting events.

Cafeteria Atmosphere

FROM DRAB TO DELIGHTFUL With effort and creativity, the school cafeteria can become a bright and cheery place to eat. Some ideas:

• Paint can do wonders for the cafeteria. Replace drab, boring walls with blocks of bright colors. Or invite the art teacher or a guest artist to coordinate students in the design and painting of a colorful cafeteria mural. (A food theme would be especially nice!)

• Collect and frame colorful posters of food to display near the serving areas (Many of the food companies listed in Appendix B provide free posters and other materials for display).

• Encourage students to design posters for the cafeteria which depict good nutrition themes.

• Display a "nutrition corner" bulletin board which is changed regularly throughout the year. Examples of themes include the *Food Guide Pyramid*, food and fitness, how food promotes a healthy heart, how to read the *Nutrition Facts* food label, the importance of calcium in building strong bones, how breakfast fuels learning, or facts about the school meal program. Consider a nearby table with handout information for students, staff, and parents. Teachers, students, and school foodservice staff can work cooperatively to design and maintain the bulletin board throughout the year.

• Add a personal touch to the cafeteria: Spruce up the serving line with colorful garnishes, display bright vinyl tablecloths on serving tables (fabric stores are an inexpensive source of colorful vinyl), purchase or make eye-catching aprons for nutrition staff and student assistants, or occasionally put out fresh cut flowers on cafeteria tables.

TIME TO EAT Offering tasty, nutritious food in a pleasant environment is not enough, though—children must have time to eat. It sounds simple enough, yet schools pressed for instructional time frequently shortchange kids by skimping on lunch time. Shortened lunch periods, coupled with long lines and slow service, may give children as few as five minutes to eat! In some schools, students opt for sack lunches just so they can bypass the lunch line.

From the time children sit down with their tray, they should be guaranteed a minimum of 20 uninterrupted minutes to eat. More time may be required for students with certain disabilities. The same holds true for breakfast—bus and morning schedules should be adjusted to allow ample time for children eating breakfast at school.

Marketing & Education

TOOT YOUR HORN! Will Rogers once said "If you done it, it ain't braggin." Many school nutrition operators would do well to brag more, spreading the *good* news about their programs. Students, teachers, and parents may not know, for instance, that the "chicken nuggets" printed on the menu are actually a low fat product or that the dinner rolls contain 50% whole wheat flour or that a fruit and vegetable bar is available daily. They may be unaware of point-of-choice nutrition information in the cafeteria or special promotions or classroom nutrition lessons taught by nutrition staff.

Effectively communicating your message is an essential ingredient to marketing success. The first step is to define your target markets. This could include the children you serve, school personnel (teachers, staff, administrators), or the community (parents, school board, media). Next, devise ways to reach these groups with your message. The examples below highlight techniques for publicizing the school meal program.

• Start with the menu. An already familiar piece, the menu adorns refrigerators each month throughout the school community. Reserve space on the *front* of the menu for nutrition tidbits, program highlights, and announcements for special promotions. Use words that denote nutrition to describe foods offered on menus, i.e. "whole grain" rolls, "lowfat" dressing, "garden fresh" broccoli florets, or "oven-baked" chicken.

Think about the design of the menu, too. Avoid using the same standard format month after month. Use computer graphics to enhance the design of the menu or enlist the help of school staff (art teachers, district graphic artists and typesetters), if available. (For more on menu design, a must-read is *Menus With Punch*, by John Bennett, *School Food Service Journal*, March 1994).

• Become an integral part of the school environment. School foodservice staff should take a keen interest in the events and programs in their school. Participate in monthly staff meetings, contribute items to the school newsletter, or volunteer to assist teachers with food and nutrition lesson planning.

• Be proactive by inviting parents, the school board, or the media to eat school breakfast or lunch. Highlight the nutrition messages and healthful choices served each day in the cafeteria. Send out notices of special promotions, contests, and events.

• Don't let national press coverage about the downside of school meals mar your program. Prepare a "fact sheet" which highlights your mission, statistics about those you serve, and a summary of positive outcomes. Send a press release to local media which emphasizes how your program offers healthful choices as well as nutrition education.

BECOME A PARTNER IN EDUCATION The nutrition concepts taught in the classroom can effectively be reinforced in the cafeteria. Beyond a health-promoting menu, school foodservice providers can also participate in nutrition education through a variety of practices, activities, and promotions:

Merchandise Healthy Foods Make sure healthful food choices beg to be eaten. The use of baskets, attractive arrangements, colorful food choices, and garnishes will make nutritious foods stand out.

Point-of-Choice Nutrition Information Display a simple nutrition analysis of foods commonly served in the cafeteria. (Consider working with a fourth or fifth grade class on determining and displaying the information.)

Include the analysis for calories, fat, carbohydrate, protein, cholesterol and sodium. Especially meaningful are comparisons of different forms of the same food such as 1% vs. 2% vs. whole milk, or pepperoni vs. mushroom pizza.

Consider highlighting other nutrients from time to time, complemented by informative posters, bulletin boards, and handouts. Examples include iron, fiber, B vitamins, or calcium.

100% Participation You can achieve complete participation—one classroom at a time, that is. Once a month, set up a "make your own lunch" bar in a chosen classroom. Students will learn basic food preparation skills as they assemble their own meal. Food bars that work particularly well include a setup for submarine or pita-pocket sandwiches, chef salads, french bread pizza topped with vegetables, or healthy nachos (made from reduced-fat corn chips, various beans, lean ground beef or ground turkey, lowfat cheese, salsa, olives, tomatoes, peppers, onions, & lowfat plain yogurt). Cover and label each student's lunch to be passed out when they come through the serving line. (Or, if you have time, coordinate the activity right before their scheduled lunch period.)

If possible, make a lunch date with each classroom in the school over the course of the year. Besides being a great opportunity for nutrition education, this activity is also a powerful way to market the school meal program to students.

Promotions and Events Make the cafeteria a fun place to learn with special promotions and thematic menus. "New Food Days" or "Food of the Week" events can feature small incentives for students who select a new healthful food. Menu, recipe, or poster contests, nutrition bingo cards, and breakfast ticket raffles are all fun ways to teach nutrition and promote the school meal program.

Posters, suggested menus, and other resources are available for specific events such as National School Lunch Week (available through the American School Food Service Association) or National Nutrition Month (sponsored by the American Dietetic Association). There are also a multitude of other special holidays and months, celebrating everything from grandparents to pickles to potatoes to heart health!

Teaching Students Many of the suggested nutrition activities and lessons described in chapters 4-11 could easily be presented by school food and nutrition professionals. Nearly every chapter includes lesson ideas that interface with the cafeteria (identified by the cafeteria icon).

Inviting classes to tour the school or central kitchen is a memorable way to introduce students to the school nutrition operation. To enhance the experience, combine the tour with a brief lesson on nutrition, give students the opportunity to plan a menu, set up a taste test for a new product, or challenge students to find a food from each food group.

School nutrition staff can also assist in career education, highlighting the job requirements and tasks of jobs such as cook, baker, chef, truck driver, school nutrition director, registered dietitian, or food technologist.

APPENDIX A

GUIDELINES FOR SAFE CLASSROOM COOKING

"I liked how you served the food with your gloves. My Mom asked if anyone touched the food."–Jenny

With so many hands busy at work, classroom cooking poses a challenge for keeping food sanitary and working conditions safe. When planning cooking projects, be sure to enlist the help of school staff or parent volunteers. The reminders below are essential for a safe, enjoyable cooking experience:

Before You Begin

• Send a letter home to parents explaining that the class will periodically participate in cooking projects which enhance the curriculum. *Be sure to elicit information on food allergies or intolerances, or any specific medical conditions that prohibit their child from eating certain foods!* Include permission slips for parents to sign and return.

• Call the local health department to find out how to become certified as a food handler. You may be required to take a course or pass a test before handling food in a public setting (local and state regulations vary).

• Be sure that all staff and volunteers who assist with classroom cooking have read and understand the guidelines presented here.

Proper Handwashing is Vital!

• Demonstrate to students the techniques for proper handwashing. Thoroughly scrub all surfaces of the hands and nails with soap, rinse with warm water, and dry with clean paper towels.

• The factor most important in producing clean hands is time. Encourage students to scrub hands for the duration of the "A-B-C song" (about 30 seconds).

• If the restroom is used for handwashing prior to handling food, prop the door open. Otherwise, students will touch the bacteria-covered doorknob on their way out.

• Remind students to wash hands after using the restroom, touching their face, hair, or neighbor, blowing their nose or sneezing, and after handling raw meat, chicken, eggs, or fish.

🖐 Tie in the concept of handwashing with a science lesson about bacteria and viruses. One kit that is especially helpful is the *Germ Buster Kit*, which uses a UV light and special soap to reveal whether hands contain "germs" (similar to the way dental disclosing tablets reveal the presence of plaque). It is available through Brevis Corporation, 3310 South 2700 East, Salt Lake City, Ut, 84109; 1-800-383-3377.

Another useful activity is to culture various surfaces such as hands, tables, or doorknobs and grow on a nutrient-rich medium in a petri dish. Once the experiment is completed, petri dishes should be rinsed with a bleach solution and carefully disposed of.

Provide a Sanitary Work Surface for Handling Food

• Desks or tables should be cleared, cleaned, and covered with clean butcher paper or a vinyl placemat/tablecloth. Cutting boards should be cleaned with hot soapy water and a sanitizing solution such as diluted bleach. (To make the bleach solution, mix 1 tablespoon institutional-strength bleach or 2 tablespoons household bleach per gallon of water.)

• Wash and sanitize all work surfaces, cutting boards, and utensils after they have come into contact with raw meat, fish, poultry, or eggs.

Emphasize Safety With Knives and Equipment

• Before allowing children to begin work on food projects, demonstrate the proper use of knives and equipment. Advise students to always cut towards their table or desk and away from their hands.

• Any equipment, even plastic serrated knives, toothpicks, or wooden skewers, can be dangerous if handled improperly. Promptly remove students who are behaving in a reckless manner with tools or equipment.

• Always use two potholders when removing foods from the microwave or oven. Be sure to turn off the stove, oven, electric fry pan, etc. when you are done cooking. Avoid knocking hot pots off the stove by turning pot and pan handles inward.

Organizing Cooking Projects

• For projects that students will prepare individually at their desk, assign three or four adult volunteers and/or students to hand out food and utensils. Those passing out supplies should practice good hygiene and always wear clean plastic gloves.

• One way to efficiently run a classroom cooking project is to organize an assembly line. Using a long table, line up the ingredients for such items as bagel pizzas, rolled burritos, stuffed pita sandwiches, or fruit-yogurt parfaits. If you utilize this method, make sure there is at least one adult at the beginning and end of the line. Just before starting through the line, students should put on clean plastic gloves.

• Time your projects so that foods do not sit at room temperature for more than two hours. The "danger zone" for rapid bacterial growth is between 40-140 degrees fahrenheit, i.e. room temperature. Pick up foods from the kitchen right before you begin the project and return leftovers upon completion. Do not allow students to "save" perishable foods to eat later in the day.

• Don't sample food products prepared with raw eggs. Even one tasty spoonful of cookie batter could harbor dangerous bacteria. Recipes that call for raw eggs, such as eggnog or homemade ice milk, should use an egg substitute which has been pasteurized.

APPENDIX B

SELECTED RESOURCES

NOTE: Some companies and organizations are listed under more than one heading.

Audiovisual Resources

The following companies feature a wide variety of resources including slides, videotapes, books, posters, computer software, and props.

FOODPLAY
    221 Pine Street
    Northampton, MA 01060
    1-800-FOODPLAY
    *Ask for information on the Emmy-award winning video
    "Janey Junkfood's Fresh Adventure."*

Lowfat Lifeline — Health Education Resources Catalog
    Valerie Parker, M.S.
    P.O. Box 1889
    Port Townsend, WA 98368
    360/379-9724
    FAX: 360/385-6835

NASCO Nutrition Teaching Aids Catalog
    901 Janesville Avenue
    P.O. Box 901
    Fort Atkinson, WI 53538-0901
    1-800-558-9595
    FAX: 414/563-8296

National Health Video
    12021 Wilshire Blvd., Suite 550
    Los Angeles, CA 90025
    1-800-543-6803
    FAX: 310/476-0503

NCES (Nutrition Counseling & Education Service) Catalog
  Patricia Stein, R.D.
  1904 E. 123rd
  Olathe, KS 66061
  1-800-445-5653

Body Image/Nutrition

Am I Fat? Helping Young Children Accept Differences in Body Size
  by Joanne Ikeda and Priscilla Naworski
  ETR Associates, 1992

How to Get Your Kid to Eat...But Not Too Much
  by Ellyn Satter
  Bull Publishing, 1987

Books For Children

See index entry "Books, Children" for a list of all children's books referenced throughout this book (coded by reading level).

Computer Programs

CD-ROM:

Dr. Health'nstein's BodyFun
  StarPress Multimedia
  303 Sacramento Street, 2nd Floor
  San Francisco, CA 94111
  1-800-782-7944

5-A-Day Adventures
  Dole Food Company, Inc.
  Nutrition Program
  155 Bovet, Suite 476
  San Mateo, CA 94402
  1-800-472-8777, ext. 555
  Send a request on school letterhead for a low-cost copy of this program aimed at third graders

Pyramid Explorer – Nutrition Adventures
  Nutrition Education Services/Oregon Dairy Council
  10505 S.W. Barbur Blvd.
  Portland, OR 97219
  (503) 229-5033

NOTE: Computer software titles for children are also listed in many of the catalogs under the *Audiovisual Resources* heading on page 163.

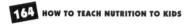

Cookbooks for Kids

American Heart Association KIDS' Cookbook
>Edited by Mary Winston
>Times Books, 1993

Come Cook With Me: A Cookbook For Kids
>by Carolyn Coats and Pamela Smith
>Carolyn Coats' Bestsellers, 1989
>(Write P.O. Box 560532, Orlando, FL 332856)

Just For Kids
>by Jen Bays Avis and Kathy F. Ward
>Avis and Ward Nutrition, Inc., 1990
>(Write 200 Professional Drive, West Monroe, LA 71291)

kids' KITCHEN: Making Good Eating Great Fun for Kids!
>by Barbara Storper
>FOODPLAY PRODUCTIONS, 1992
>*(See page 163 for address)*

Kitchen Fun For KIDS
>by Michael Jacobson and Laura Hill
>Henry Holt and Company, New York, 1991

The Healthy Start Kids' Cookbook: Fun and Healthful Recipes That Kids Can Make Themselves
>Edited by Sandra K. Nissenberg
>Chronimed, 1994

The Multicultural Cookbook for Students
>by Carole Lisa Albyn and Lois Sinaiko Webb
>Oryx Press, 1993.
>*Written for intermediate and secondary students, this book is nevertheless an excellent resource for primary students and teachers studying about the food culture of various countries.*

The Science Chef: 100 Fun Food Experiments and Recipes for Kids
>by Joan D'Amico and Karen Eich Drummond
>John Wiley & Sons, 1995

Young Chefs Nutrition Guide and Cookbook
>by Carolyn Moore, Mimi Kerr, and Robert Shulman
>Barron's Publishing, 1990

Fitness

For Adults Working With Children:

Fitness for Kids Ages 6-10: A Guide to Health, Exercise, & Nutrition
by Arnold Schwarzenegger with Charles Gaines
Doubleday, 1993

Play Hard, Eat Right: A Parent's Guide to Sports Nutrition for Children
by Debbi S. Jennings and Suzanne N. Steen
Chronimed, 1995

For Kids:

SPORTSWORKS: More than 50 fun activities that explore the science of sport
by the Ontario Science Centre
Addison-Wesley, 1989

Organizations Providing Fitness Resources:

American Alliance of Health, Physical Education,
Recreation and Dance (AAHPERD)
1900 Association Drive
Reston, VA 22091
Write for information on the "Physical Best" program.

The President's Council on Physical Fitness and Sports
701 Pennsylvania Avenue, NW
Washington, DC 20004
Write for information on the "President's Challenge" fitness test, the free booklet "Get Fit," and "The President's Youth Fitness Program".

Food Companies/Commissions

Food companies and commissions are often a great source for low-cost posters, flyers, recipes and nutrition education curricula.

A WORD OF CAUTION: Please read all company-sponsored materials carefully before using with students. Some materials may read like an advertisement or contain biased information. Choose materials that present a balanced view of nutrition.

The American Institute of Wine and Food
1550 Bryant Street
7th Floor
San Francisco, CA 94103
AIWF has the free program, "Sensory Sleuths", which is designed to teach children how to use sight, touch, sound, smell, and taste to help determine food choices.

California Apricot Advisory Board
1280 Blvd Way
Walnut Creek, CA 94595

California Egg Commission
c/o The Londre Company, Inc.
3393 Barham Blvd, First Floor
Los Angeles, CA 90068

California Kiwi Fruit Commission
1540 River Park Drive, Suite 110
Sacramento, CA 95815

California Strawberry Advisory Board
PO Box 269
Watsonville, CA 95076

California Table Grape Commission
PO Box 5498
Fresno, CA 93755

Dole Food Service
PO Box 810
Hudson, WI 54016

Dry Pea and Lentil Industries
Stateline Office
Moscow, ID 83843
> *Request the pamphlet "Legume Your Menu" and the "Nutrition and You" curriculum.*

Florida Department of Citrus
PO Box 148
Lakeland, FL 33802

Idaho Bean Commission
PO Box 9433
Boise, ID 83707

International Apple Institute
PO Box 1137
McLean, VA 22101
> *Request information on the "Gimme Five" curriculum.*

International Food Information Council (IFIC) Foundation
1100 Connecticut Avenue, N.W.
Suite 430
Washington, DC 20036
> *Publishes a variety of free materials that address children's nutrition. Ask for a free "Publications List."*

Kellogg Company
Battle Creek, MI 49016
> *Request a free copy of the "FIT TO BE" video.*

National Dairy Council
10255 West Higgins Road, Ste. 900
Rosemont, IL 60018
> *Publishes extensive nutrition education materials for all ages. Ask for a free catalog. (For best results, contact your state Dairy Council or Associated Milk Producers office)*

National Livestock and Meat Board
444 N. Michigan Avenue
Chicago, IL 60611

Northwest Cherry Growers
1005 Tieton Drive
Yakima, WA 98902

Oregon Dairy Council/Nutrition Education Services
10505 SW Barbur Blvd
Portland, OR 97219
Not affiliated with National Dairy Council. Publishes an excellent collection of nutrition education resources.

Oregon-Washington California Pear Bureau
813 SW Alder, Suite 601
Portland, OR 97205-3182

Peanut Advisory Board
1950 North Park Place, Suite 525
Atlanta, GA 30339

Rice Council of America
PO Box 22802
Houston, TX 77027

Sunkist Growers, Inc.
PO Box 7888
Van Nuys, CA 91409

The National Potato Board
1385 S Colorado Blvd, #512
Denver, CO 80222

The Sugar Association
1101 15th Street, NW, Suite 600
Washington, DC 20005

Washington Apple Commission
PO Box 550
Wenatchee, WA 98807
Ask for information on the "Healthy Choices for Kids" curriculum.

Food Models

NASCO Nutrition Teaching Aids Catalog
    901 Janesville Avenue
    PO Box 901
    Fort Atkinson, WI 53538-0901
    1-800-558-9595
    FAX: 414/563-8296
    NASCO offers a large assortment of food models constructed from soft vinyl plastic.

National Dairy Council
10255 West Higgins Road, Ste. 900
Rosemont, IL 60018
    A low-cost source of life-sized, punch-out food photographs. The back of each model includes nutrient information. (For best results, contact your state Dairy Council or Associated Milk Producers office)

Food Guide Pyramid

Consumer Information Center
Department 159-Y
Pueblo, CO 81009
    To order a copy of "The Food Guide Pyramid" booklet, send a $1.00 check made out to the Superintendent of Documents. Include a request for a Food Guide Pyramid poster.

National Livestock and Meat Board
Education Department
444 N. Michigan Avenue
Chicago, IL 60611
    Send a request on school letterhead for a free or low-cost classroom-sized Food Guide Pyramid poster.

PYRAMID POWER
Cooperative Extension in Lancaster County
444 Cherrycreek Road
Lincoln, NE 68528-1507
    Pyramid Power is a bingo-type nutrition game that reinforces the concepts of the Food Guide Pyramid.

U.S. Department of Agriculture
Human Nutrition Information Service
6505 Belcrest Road
Hyattsville, MD 20782

> *Write for a free copy of Nutrition and Your Health: Dietary Guidelines For Americans, HG-232. Be sure and ask for a list of all nutrition materials published by USDA, including those which feature the Food Guide Pyramid.*

Washington State Dairy Council
4201 – 198th St. S.W. Suite 102
Lynnwood, WA 98036
PHONE: (206) 744-1616; Toll Free FAX: 1-800-470-1222

> *Write for information on how to order bright, colorful Food Guide Pyramid stickers. Stickers depicting each individual food group as well as the pyramid in its entirety are available.*

Young People's Healthy Heart Program
Mercy Hospital
570 Chautauqua Boulevard
Valley City, ND 58072

> *Publishes Food Guide Pyramid lesson plans and games for different levels.*

Gardening

Children's Seed Program
Brooklyn Botanic Garden
1000 Washington Avenue
Brooklyn, NY 1122501099

> *This program offers reasonably priced seeds and gardening supplies for children and beginning gardeners.*

GrowLab
National Gardening Association
180 Flynn Avenue
Burlington, VT 05401
1-800-538-7476

> *The GrowLab program is a comprehensive, science-based curriculum for grades K-8. The program features indoor gardening equipment, books, posters, videos, and curricula.*

Let's Get Growing!
1900 Commercial Way
Santa Cruz, CA 95065
> This catalog offers a wide variety of curricula, kits, and garden-based science supplies for the classroom.

Life Lab Science Program
1156 High Street
Santa Cruz, CA 95064
> *The award winning Life Lab Science program is a grade-specific, core curriculum of garden-based science. "The Growing Classroom" is a supplemental activity guide which contains a number of nutrition-related activities.*

Washington State University
Pierce County Cooperative Extension
3049 S 36th Street, Suite 300
Tacoma, WA 98409
> *WSU publishes the program "Growing With Plants," a first-second grade curriculum blending plant science, nutrition, and ecology.*

Garnishing

The following books include colorful photographs and helpful illustrations on creating garnishes.

Fun Foods: Clever Ideas for Garnishing & Decorating
> by Wim Kros
> Sterling Publishing Co., 1990

Garnishing: A Feast for Your Eyes
> by Francis Talyn Lynch
> HP Books, 1987

How to Garnish
> by Harvey Rosen
> International Culinary Consultants, 1983

Melon Garnishing
> by Harvey Rosen
> International Culinary Consultants, 1983

General Reference

Bowes & Church's Food Values of Portions Commonly Used
  16th edition
  by Jean A.T. Pennington
  J.B. Lippincott, 1993
  Aimed at nutrition professionals, this is the definitive source for the complete nutritional breakdown of 8500 foods.

NETP (Nutrition Education & Training Program)

NETP is one component of the federal child nutrition programs. Each state has a NETP coordinator that directs the use of these nutrition education funds. Generally speaking, funds are used for training foodservice staff and classroom teachers, developing materials and resources, and providing grants for innovative school-based nutrition education initiatives. In many states, NETP is a source of free or low-cost nutrition education resources.

To find out more about NETP in your state, contact the state department of education or the state health department. NETP coordinators are most often employed within the child nutrition office but may be housed within the health or education divisions.

Nutrition Facts Food Label

Professional Resources on Food Labeling Education
Last updated in February 1996, this list from the **Food and Nutrition Information Center** (FNIC) contains nearly 100 resources on Nutrition Facts food labels. The types of resources reviewed include books, magazines, and reprints; brochures, fact sheets, and other handouts; curriculums, lesson plans, and teaching kits; posters, poster kits, and transparencies; promotional materials; slide presentations; software and exhibit materials.

The document is available on the Internet at http://www.nal.usda.gov/fnic/pubs/gen/labprobr.htm. or contact FNIC at the address below.

Food and Nutrition Information Center
Agricultural Research Service, USDA
National Agricultural Library, Room 304
10301 Baltimore Avenue
Beltsville, MD 20705-2351
301-504-5719
FAX: 301-504-6856
email: fnic@nal.usda.gov

Organizations

American Cancer Society
1599 Clifton Road, NE
Atlanta, GA 30329
1-800-ACS-2345
> *For best results, contact your state ACS office.*

American Heart Association
National Center
7272 Greenville Avenue
Dallas, TX 75231-4596
> *For best results, contact your state affiliate.*

Center for Science in the Public Interest
1501 16th Street N.W.
Washington, D.C. 20036
> *A particularly good CSPI resource is Eat, Think, and Be Healthy: Creative Nutrition Activities for Children.*

Five a Day for Better Health Program
Cancer Prevention and Control Extramural Research Branch
National Cancer Institute
9000 Rockville Pike, EPN-330
Rockville, MD 20982
(301) 496-8520
> *Ask for "Five A Day" materials that have been developed for classroom use.*

National Center for Nutrition and Dietetics
216 W. Jackson Boulevard
Chicago, IL 60606-6995
1-800-366-1655
> *When you call the toll free hotline, you can either hear prerecorded nutrition messages or ask to speak with a registered dietitian. Ask for the most recent "Catalog of Products and Services," for materials published by The American Dietetic Association*

USDA National Agricultural Library
6th Floor, NAL Bldg.
10301 Baltimore Blvd.
Beltsville, MD 20705-2351

The NAL houses a large collection of materials and a free lending service for classroom teachers, librarians, school foodservice providers, and others associated with federal child nutrition programs. Be sure to request the bibliography "Nutrition Education Materials and Audiovisuals for Grades Preschool through 6." The library also provides articles and training materials on implementing the dietary guidelines and merchandising school food service.

Penn State Nutrition Center
417 E. Calder Way
University Park, PA 16801-5663

This center houses a collection of videos, curricula, activity kits, and computer software for use in the classroom. Write for a free catalog.

Portland Public Schools
Nutrition Services
501 N. Dixon
Portland, OR 97227

Ask for information on the "F.U.N." (Fundamental Understanding of Nutrition) and "Nutrition From the Culinary View" curricula published by PPS. (Both programs developed under the direction of this author)

Puppetry

NET Workshop Coordinator
Texas Department of Human Services
PO Box 149030 MC Y-906
Austin, TX 78714-9030
NUTRITION HOTLINE: 1-800-982-3621

Ask about the "Puppetry in Nutrition Education" workshops and available resource materials.

Paper Masks and Puppets for Stories, Songs, and Plays
    by Ron and Marsha Feller
    The Arts Factory, 1985
    (Write: PO Box 55547, Seattle, WA 98155)

Yummy Designs
    Nutrition Education Materials and Programs
    PO Box 1851
    Walla Walla, WA 99362

School Foodservice

Advocates for Better Children's Diets (ABCD) Coalition
1723 U Street, NW
Washington, DC 20009
    The ABCD coalition is comprised of companies and organizations with an interest in children's nutrition. Ask about the publication "Making the Honor Roll: A Community Action Guide to Improve Kids' Diets Through Child Nutrition Programs."

American School Food Service Association
1600 Duke Street, 7th floor
Alexandria, VA 22314-3436
    ASFSA has developed the "Healthy E.D.G.E." (Eating, the Dietary Guidelines, and Education), as a training program for school lunch providers. Members also receive the journal "School Foodservice and Nutrition" and have access to the ASFSA Emporium, a catalog of products and resources.

American Heart Association
National Center
7272 Greenville Avenue
Dallas, TX 75231-4596
    Contact your state affiliate to request information on the AHA "Hearty School Lunch" program.

American Cancer Society
1599 Clifton Road, NE
Atlanta, GA 30329
1-800-ACS-2345
    Contact your state ACS office and ask about the "Changing the Course" program.

Healthy School Meals Resource System
United States Department of Agriculture Food and Nutrition Information Center
National Agricultural Library, Room 304
10301 Baltimore Avenue
Beltsville, MD 20705-2351

This newly implemented system provides information and instructional materials that support the efforts of school nutrition personnel. Database information is available via the Internet (http://schoolmeals.nalusda.gov:8001), on disk, or written copy.

National Food Service Management Institute
PO Drawer 188
University, MS 38677-0188
1-800-321-3061

The NFSMI was established to develop and provide educational materials and training programs for school foodservice providers. Request information on training seminars and teleconferences, the free loan program for nutrition education materials, and other available resources.

National Livestock and Meat Board
Education Department
444 N. Michigan Avenue
Chicago, IL 60611

Ask for information regarding the "Lunchpower" healthy schools lunches program.

Public Voice for Food and Health Policy
1101 14th Street, N.W.
Suite 710
Washington, DC 20005

A national, nonprofit advocacy organization, Public Voice publishes an annual report on the status of school meal programs. "Serving Up Success: Schools Making Nutrition a Priority," (published August, 1994) describes 41 school districts who successfully promote a healthful menu and nutrition education.

Vegetarian Education Network
PO Box 3347
West Chester, PA 19380

A great source for vegetarian menu ideas and quantity recipes suitable for use in the school meal program.

BIBLIOGRAPHY

American Dietetic Association. Position of the American Dietetic Association: Child nutrition services. *J Am Diet Assoc.* 1993;93:334-336.

American Dietetic Association. Position of the American Dietetic Association: Competitive foods in schools. *J Am Diet Assoc.* 1991;91:1123-1125.

American Dietetic Association. School-based nutrition programs and services: Position of ADA, SNE, and ASFSA. *J Am Diet Assoc.* 1995;95:367-369.

Arbeit ML, Johnson CC, Mott DS, Harsha DW, Nicklas TA, Webber LS,

Berenson GS. The Heart Smart Cardiovascular School Health Promotion: behavior correlates of risk factor change. *Prev Med.* 1992;21:18-32.

Bennett J. Menus with punch. *School Food Ser J.* 1994;March:43-48.

Birch LL. Children's eating: are manners enough? *J Gastronomy.* 1993;7:19-25.

Britten P. Assessing the needs for nutrition education—knowledge, beliefs and practices of students, teachers and food service managers. Presentation at July 1994, Society for Nutrition Education Annual Meeting.

Burghardt J, Devaney B. The School Nutrition Dietary Assessment Study: Summary of Findings. Princeton, NJ: Mathematica Policy Research, Inc., 1993.

Chandra RK. Primary prevention of cardiovascular disease in childhood: recent knowledge and unanswered questions. *J Am Coll Nutr.* 1992;11:3S-7S.

Coddington RM. A "NAC" for excitement. *School Food Serv J.* 1995;January:45-48.

Consumers Union Education Services. *Selling America's Kids: Commercial Pressures on Kids of the 90's.* Mount Vernon, New York, 1990.

Cotugna N. TV ads on Saturday morning children's programming—what's new? *J Nutr Ed.* 1988;20:125-127.

Crockett SJ, Mullis R, Perry CL, Luepker RV. Parent education in youth-directed nutrition interventions. *Prev Med.* 1989;18:475-491.

Davis J, Oswalt R. Societal influences on a thinner body size in children. *Percept Mot Skills.* 1992;74:697-698.

Derrickson JP, Widodo MME, Jarosz LA. Providers of food to homeless and hungry people need more dairy, fruit, vegetable, and lean-meat items. *J Am Diet Assoc.* 1994;94:445-446.

Dietz WH. You are what you eat—what you eat is what you are. *J Adol Health Care.* 1990;11:76-81.

Farris RP, Nicklas TA, Webber LS, Berenson GS. Nutrient contribution of the school lunch program: implications for healthy people 2000. *J Sch Health.* 1992;62:180-184.

Fisher B, Hopper C, Munoz K. Fitting in fitness: an integrated approach to health, nutrition, and exercise. *Learning91.* 1991;July/August:25-54.

Fisher JG. How I turned my classroom into a health club. *Instructor.* 1987;March:80-81.

Food Research Action Center. *Community Childhood Hunger Identification Project: A Survey of Childhood Hunger in the United States. Executive Summary.* Washington, DC, 1991.

Fussell B. *The Story of Corn.* New York: Alfred A Knoff, 1992.

Gay, K. *Caution! This May Be An Advertisement (A Teen Guide to Advertising).* Franklin Watts, 1992.

Good Nutrition: A School Nutrition & Summer Food Service Newsletter. Eat five fruits and vegetables and call me in the morning. Oregon Department of Education, Winter 1994.

Gortmaker SL, Dietz WH, Cheung LWY. Inactivity, diet, and the fattening of America. *J Am Diet Assoc.* 1990;90:1247-1252.

Gustafson-Larson AM, Terry RD. Weight-related behaviors and concerns of fourth-grade children. *J Am Diet Assoc.* 1992;92:818-822.

Gwynn ML. A growing phenomenon. *Science and Children.* 1988;April:25-26

Harding Lawson Associates. Offer Versus Serve and Food Choices in Elementary School Cafeterias: Waste Prevention Pilot Projects at North Plains Elementary School, Charles F. Tigard Elementary School, and Metzger Elementary School, Unpublished data, May 1994.

International Food Information Council. *Kids make the nutritional grade*. New York, NY: YOUTH Research Survey, June, 1992.

International Food Information Council & The American Dietetic Association. *How are kids making food choices?* Princeton, NJ: The Gallup Organization, Inc., July, 1991.

J Sch Health. Healthy People 2000: National Health Promotion and Disease Prevention Objectives and Healthy Schools. 1991;61:298-328.

Jensen HC, Ferris AM, Neafsey PJ, Gorham RL. Promoting school lunch participation through nutrition education. *J Nutr Ed*. 1985;17:15-18.

Johnson C. Taking the classroom beyond four walls. *Newsletter of OAAHE*, Spring 1989

Kaplan RM, Toshima MT. Does a reduced fat diet cause retardation in child growth? *Prev Med*. 1992;21:33-52.

Kelder SH, Perry CL, Klepp KI, Lytle L. Longitudinal tracking of adolescent smoking, physical activity, and food choice behaviors. *Am J Public Health*. 1994;84:1121-1126.

Kellogg Company. *The Kellogg Children's Nutrition Survey. Executive Summary*. Battle Creek, Mich, 1991.

Kirks BA, Hughes, C. Long-term behavioral effects of parent involvement in nutrition education. *J Nutr Ed*. 1986;18:203-206.

Knutsen SF, Knutsen R. The Tromso survey: the family intervention study—the effect of intervention on some coronary risk factors and dietary habits, a 6-year follow-up. *Prev Med*. 1991;20:197-212.

Kotz K, Story M. Food advertisements during children's Saturday morning television programming: Are they consistent with dietary recommendations? *J Am Diet Assoc*. 1994;94:1296-1300.

Lavine SA. *Indian Corn and Other Gifts*. Dodd, Mead, & Co., 1974.

Lewis C. Healthy People 2000—Progress Review. Presentation at July 1994, Society for Nutrition Education Annual Meeting.

Lifshitz F. Children on adult diets: Is it harmful? Is it healthful? *J Am Coll Nutr*. 1992;11:84S-90S.

Mackenzie M. Is the family meal disappearing? *J Gastronomy*. 1993;7:35-45.

Mellin LM, Irwin CE, Scully S. Prevalence of disordered eating in girls: A survey of middle-class children. *J Am Diet Assoc*. 1992;92:851-853.

Mellin L. To: President Clinton Re: Combating childhood obesity. *J Am Diet Assoc*. 1993;93:265-266.

Meyers AF, Sampson AE, Weitzman M, Rogers BL, Kayne H. School breakfast program and school performance. *Am J Dis Child*. 1989;143:1234-1239.

Mintz SW. Feeding, eating, and grazing: some speculations on modern food habits. *J Gastronomy*. 1993;7:46-57.

Murphy AS, Youatt JP, Hoerr SL, Sawyer CA, Andrews SL. Nutrition education needs and learning preferences of Michigan students in grades 5, 8 and 11. *J Sch Health*. 1994:64:273-278.

National Cholesterol Education Program Expert Panel on Blood Cholesterol Levels in Children and Adolescents. Highlights of the report of the expert panel on blood cholesterol levels in children and adolescents. *Am Fam Physician*. 1992;45:2127-2136.

National Education Association. *The Relationship Between Nutrition and Learning*. Alexandria, VA, 1990.

Nelson CJ. Harvesting a curriculum. *Science and Children*. 1988;April:22-24.

Nestle M. School lunch: A key to improved nutrition. *School Food Ser J*. 1991;August:33-34.

Nicklas TA, Bao W, Webber LS, Berenson GS. Breakfast consumption affects adequacy of total daily intake in children. *J Am Diet Assoc*. 1993;93:886-891.

Nicklas TA, Webber LS, Srinivasan SR, Berenson GS. Secular trends in dietary intakes and cardiovascular risk factors of 10-y-old children: The Bogalusa Heart Study (1973-1988). *Am J Clin Nutr*. 1993;57:930-937.

NIH Consensus Development Panel on Optimal Calcium Intake. Optimal calcium intake. *J Am Med Assoc*. 1994;272:1942-1948.

Nitzke S. Opportunities and challenges for school-based nutrition education. Presentation at July 1994, Society for Nutrition Education Annual Meeting.

Olson CM, Frongillo EA, Schardt DG. Status of nutrition education in elementary schools: 1981 vs. 1975. *J Nutr Ed*. 1986;18:49-54.

PDAY Research Group. Natural history of aortic and coronary atherosclerotic lesions in youth: Findings from the PDAY study. *Arterioscler Thromb*. 1993;13:1291-1298.

Perry CL, Luepker RV, Murray DM, Kurth C, Mullis R, Crockett S, Jacobs DR. Parent involvement with children's health promotion: The Minnesota home team. *Am J Public Health*. 1988;78:1156-1160.

Perry CL, Stone EJ, Parcel GS, Ellison RC, Nader PR, Webber LS, Luepker RV. School-based cardiovascular health promotion: the child and adolescent trial for cardiovascular health (CATCH). *J Sch Health*. 1990;60:406-413.

Pierce JW, Wardle J. Self-esteem, parental appraisal and body size in children. *J Child Psychol Psychiatry*. 1993;34:1125-1136.

POST Center for Nutrition & Health. Consumer survey on questions Americans most want answered about nutrition as it relates to health. White Plains, NY. May, 1989.

Rossow I, Rise J. Concordance of parental and adolescent health behaviors. *Soc Sci Med*. 1994;38:1299-1305.

Russo, LA. Practices and opinions of Wisconsin elementary school teachers regarding nutrition education. Presentation at July 1994, Society for Nutrition Education Annual Meeting.

Sampson AE, Meyers A, Rogers BL, Weitzman M. School breakfast program participation and parental attitudes. *J Nutr Ed*. 1991;23:110-115.

Schlicker SA, Borra ST, Regan C. The weight and fitness status of United States children. *Nutr Rev*. 1994;52:11-17.

School Food Ser J. Study challenges Saturday morning advertisers. 1991;August:20.

Serdula MK, Ivery D, Coates RJ, Freedman DS, Williamson DF, Byers T. Do obese children become obese adults? A review of the literature. *Prev Med*. 1993;22:167-177.

Shannon B, Peacock J, Brown MJ. Body fatness, television viewing and calorie-intake of a sample of Pennsylvania sixth grade children. *J Nutr Ed*. 1991;23:262-268.

Simons-Morton BG, Parcel GS, Baranowski T, Forthofer R, O'Hara NM. Promoting physical activity and a healthful diet among children: results of a school-based intervention study. *Am J Public Health*. 1991;81:986-991.

Stefkovich C. The value of diversity. School Food Serv Nutr. 1994;October:61-63.

Taras HL, Sallis JF, Patterson TL, Nader PR, Nelson JA. Television's influence on children's diet and physical activity. *J Dev Behav Pediatr*. 1989;10:176-180.

Thomas LF, Long EM, Zaske JM. Nutrition education sources and priorities of elementary school teachers. *J Am Diet Assoc*. 1994;94:318-320.

Center on Hunger, Poverty, and Nutrition Policy. *The Link Between Nutrition and Cognitive Development in Children*. Tufts University School of Nutrition, 1994.

U.S. Department of Agriculture/U.S. Department of Health and Human Services. *Nutrition and Your Health: Dietary Guidelines for Americans, 3rd ed*. Washington, DC: U.S. Government Printing Office, Home and Garden Bulletin No. 232, 1990.

U.S. Department of Agriculture/Human Nutrition Information Service. *The Food Guide Pyramid*. Home and Garden Bulletin No. 252, 1992.

Weiss EH, Kien CL. A synthesis of research on nutrition education at the elementary school level. *J Sch Health*. 1987;57:8-12.

Whitaker RC, Wright JA, Koepsell TD, Finch AJ, Psaty BM. Randomized intervention to increase children's selection of low-fat foods in school lunches. *J Pediatr*. 1994;125:535-540.

Williams MH. Exercise effects on children's health. *Sports Science Exchange*. Chicago, IL: The Gatorade Sports Science Institute, March 1993.

Wolfe WS, Campbell CC. Food pattern, diet quality, and related characteristics of schoolchildren in New York State. *J Am Diet Assoc*. 1993;93:1280-1284.

Wolfe WS, Campbell CC, Frongillo EA, Haas JD, Melnik TA. Overweight schoolchildren in New York State: prevalence and characteristics. *Am J Public Health*. 1994;84:807-813.

INDEX

ORDER FORM

To order additional copies of HOW TO TEACH NUTRITION TO KIDS, send payment to:

Connie Evers

24 Carrot Press

P.O. Box 23546 • Tigard, OR 97281-3546

Quantity discounts are available. Call for rates.

Phone/Fax: (503)524-9318 • email: eversc@ohsu.edu

HOW TO TEACH NUTRITION TO KIDS: An integrated, creative approach to nutrition education for children ages 6-10

_____ copies at $18.00 per copy $ _____

Shipping & Handling ($2.50 per book) $ _____

TOTAL ENCLOSED $ _____

Name_____

Address_____

City _____ State _____ Zip _____

Telephone _____ Fax _____ Email _____

MasterCard/VISA #_____ Exp. Date _____

Authorizing Signature _____

HOW TO TEACH NUTRITION TO KIDS: An integrated, creative approach to nutrition education for children ages 6-10

_____ copies at $18.00 per copy $ _____

Shipping & Handling ($2.50 per book) $ _____

TOTAL ENCLOSED $ _____

Name_____

Address_____

City _____ State _____ Zip _____

Telephone _____ Fax _____ Email _____

MasterCard/VISA #_____ Exp. Date _____

Authorizing Signature _____